Marie Tanneux

Illustrations by Lili la baleine

Translated by Dipa Chaudhuri

AF654154

Three little pigs

A tale along with postures on shaping up well

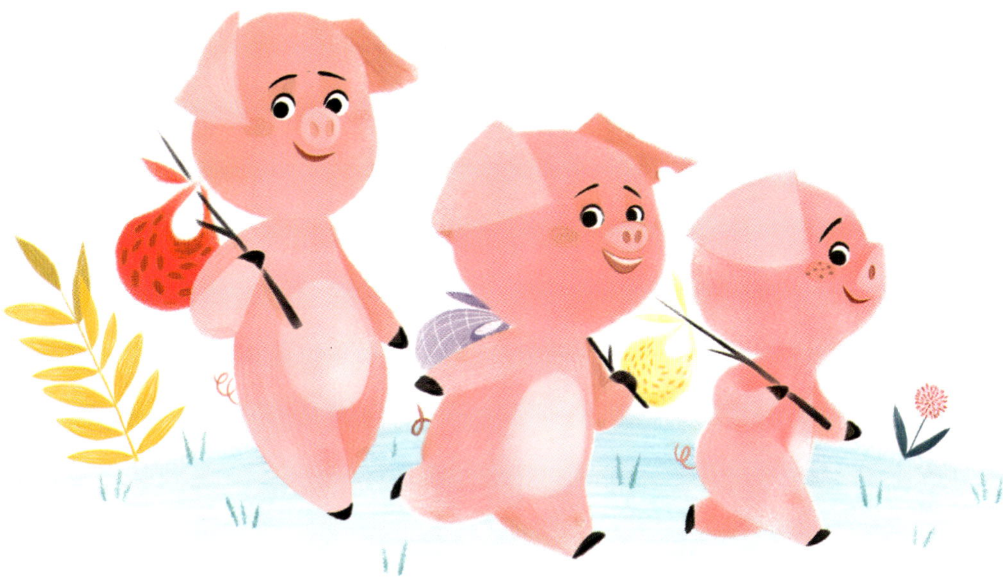

Om Books International

Listening

To start with, get ready to listen to the story.

Benefit: This posture helps the child focus.

5 breaths

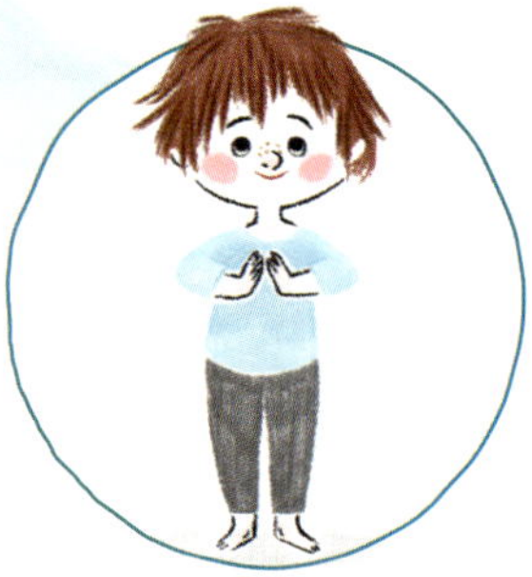

While standing, join your hands in front of your chest and bow your head.

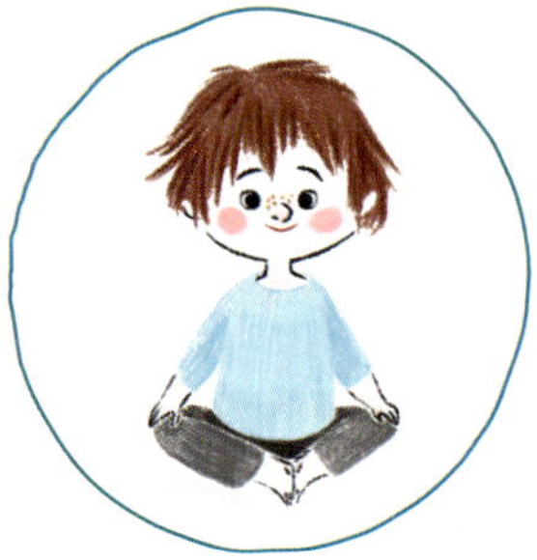

Sit down, with your back straight and your legs crossed.

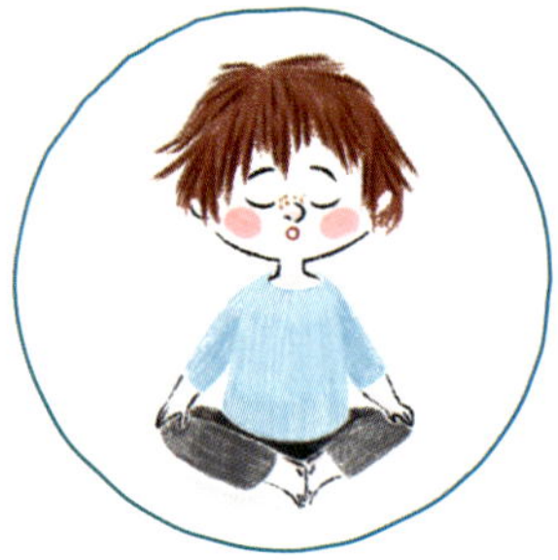

Breathe deep. Close your eyes. You are ready to listen to the story.

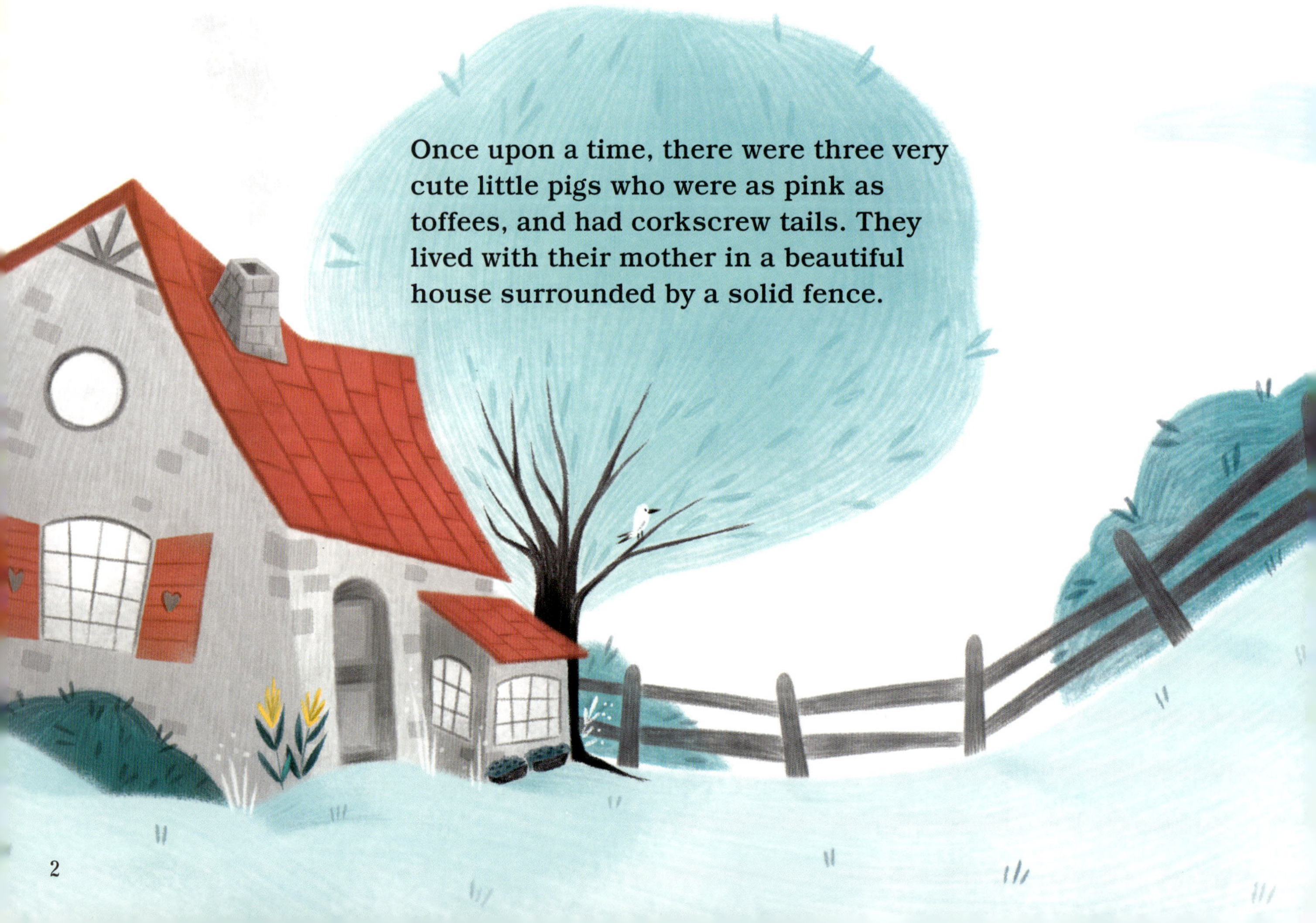

Once upon a time, there were three very cute little pigs who were as pink as toffees, and had corkscrew tails. They lived with their mother in a beautiful house surrounded by a solid fence.

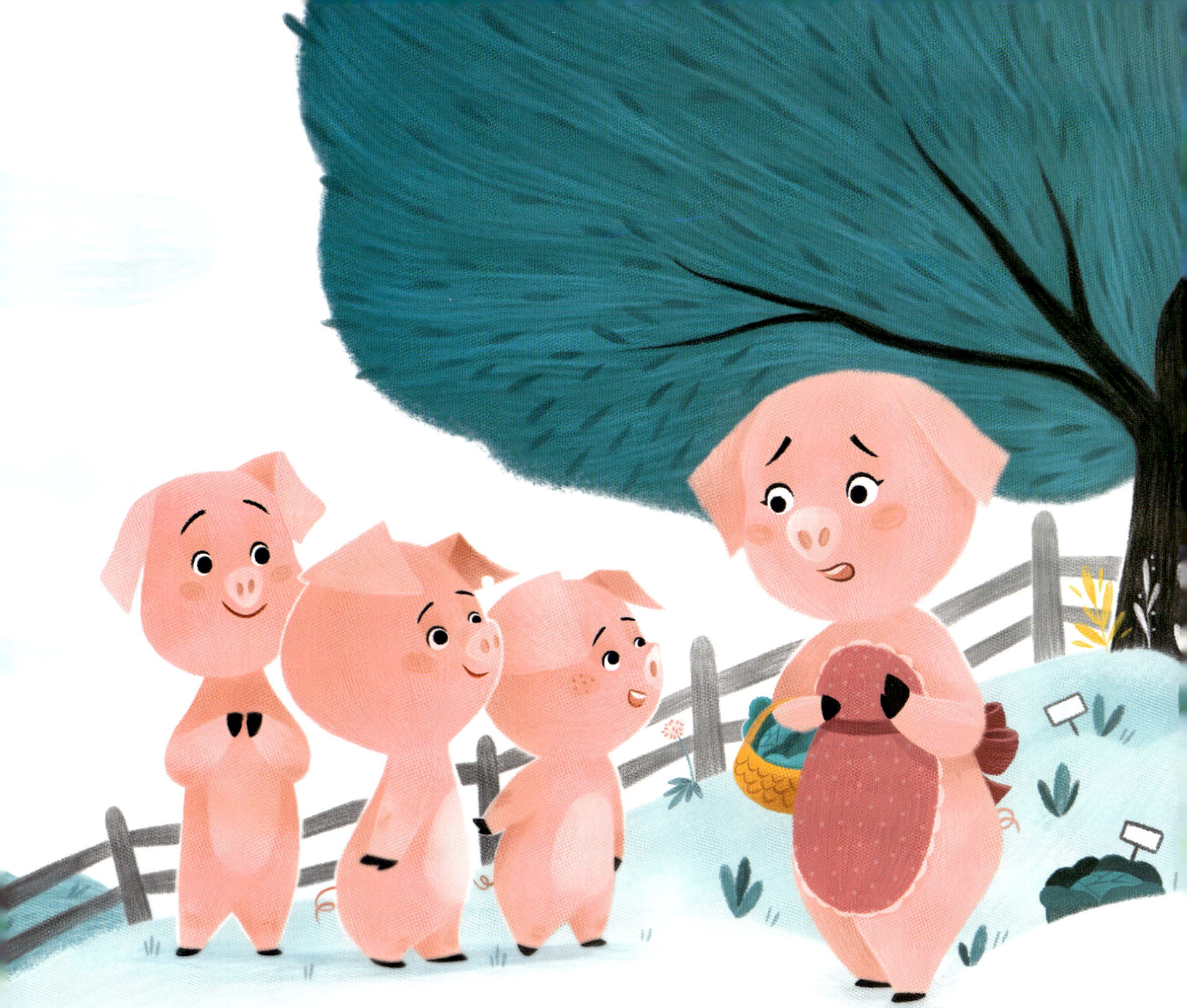

One day, they said to their mother:
“We want to leave, discover nature and live in the forest.
“In the forest? But there are so many dangers lurking in it!
“And the fox could well catch you and gobble you up!” said the mother of the three little pigs.

But since they were determined to live in the forest, their mother let them go. After exchanging a hundred kisses, a thousand suggestions and the promise to construct solid houses, they prepared their backpack and left, whistling.

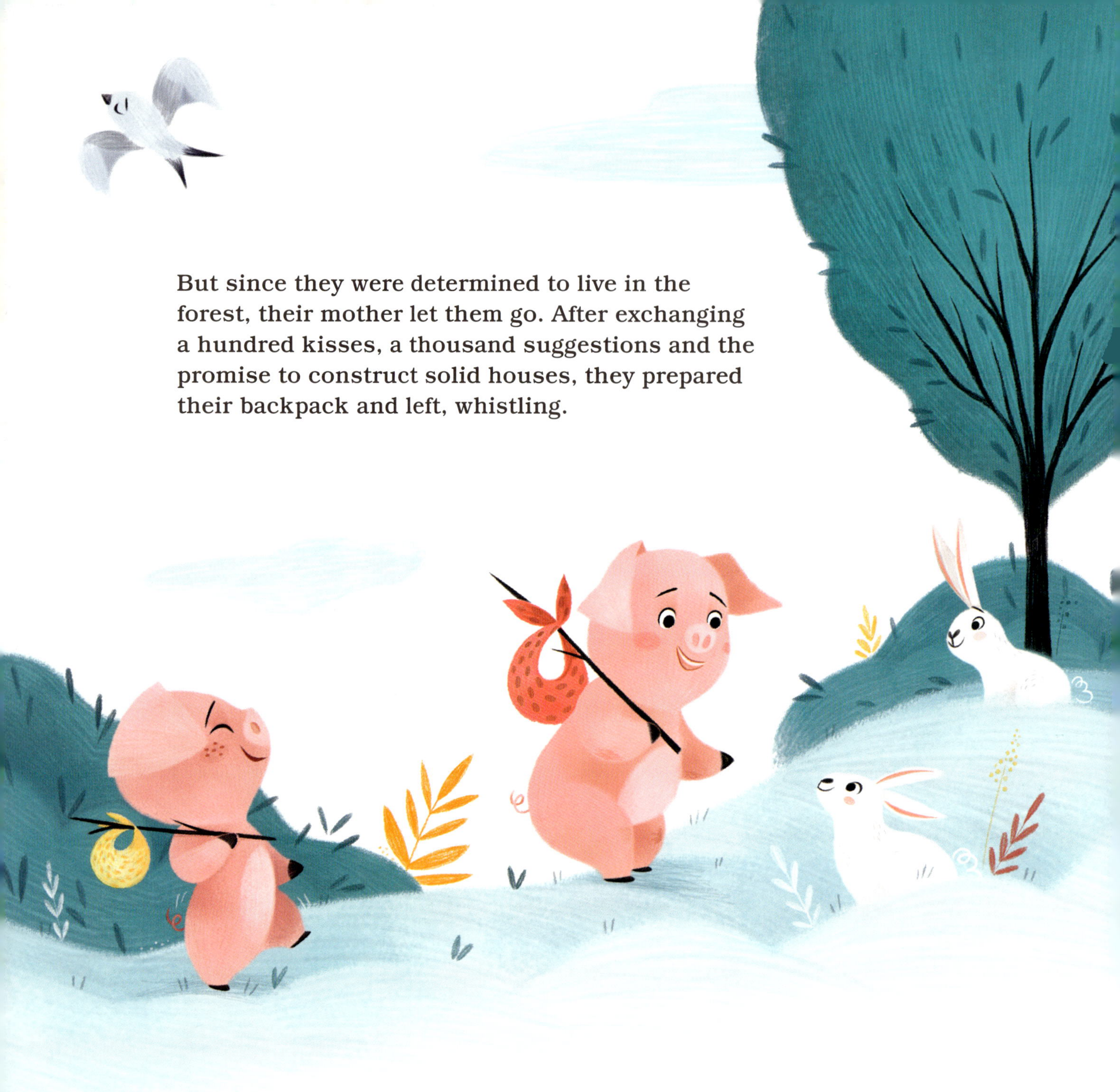

After a long walk, they finally arrived in the forest.

How enchanting! It was bathed in sunlight and birdsong. The animals came out to greet them and play with them.

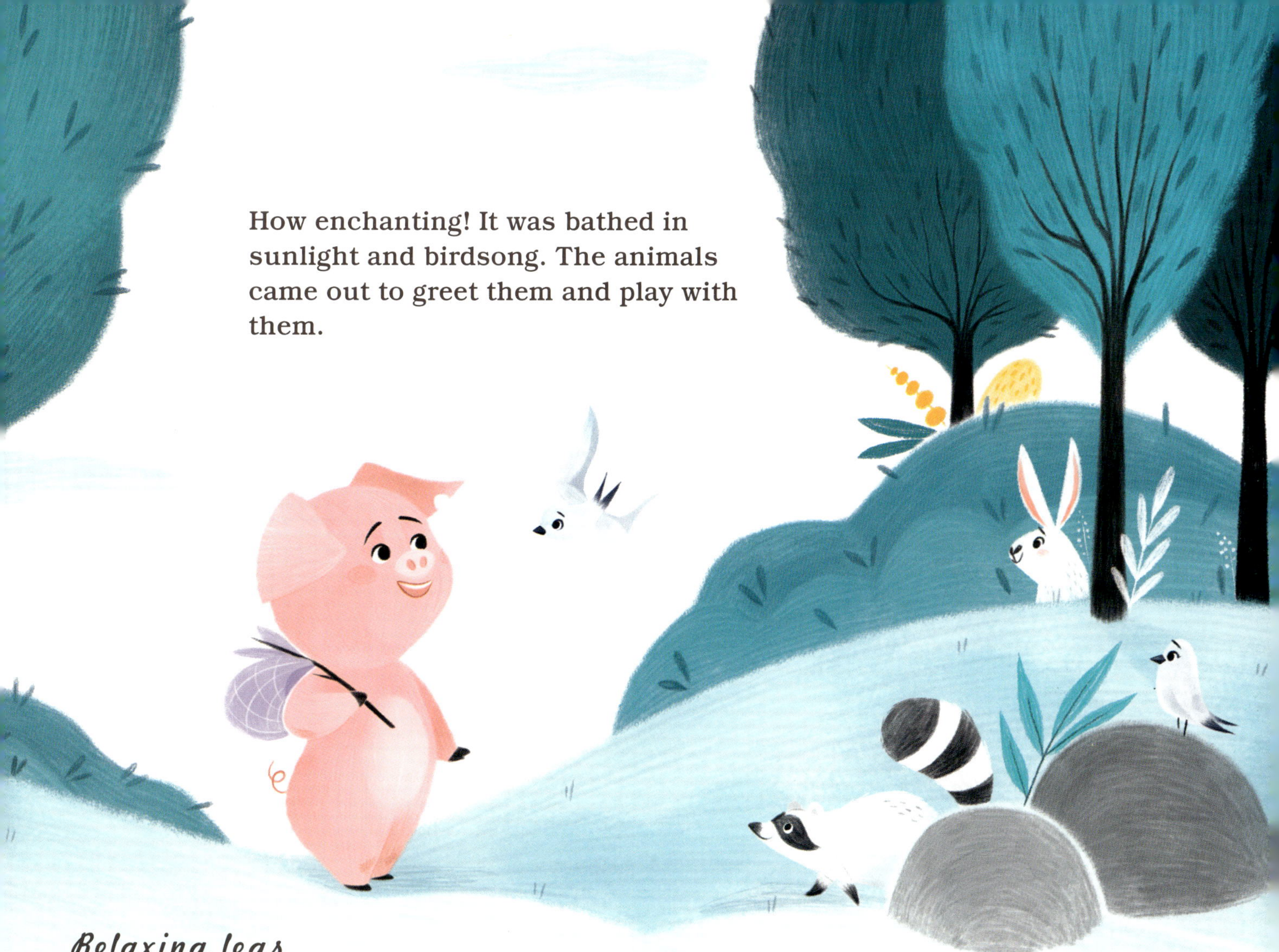

Relaxing legs

The three brothers have walked for a long time. It is time to relax the legs.

Benefits: This movement is good for calm and balance

10 times

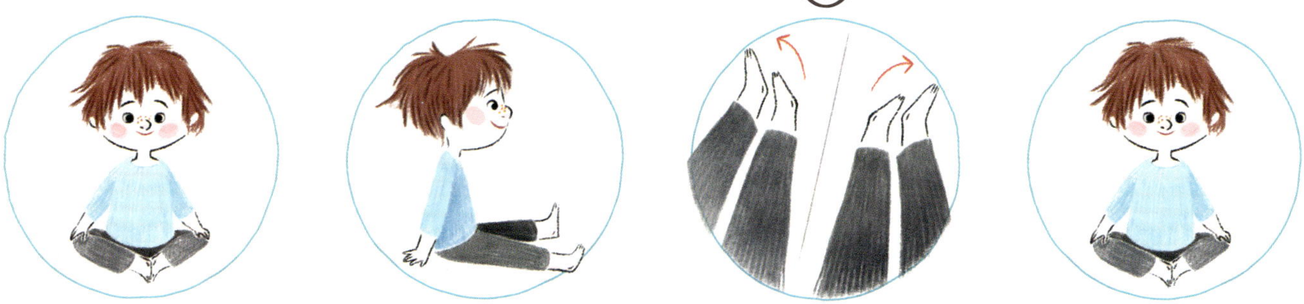

Sit cross-legged, with your back straight.	Place your legs slightly apart in a relaxed manner in front of you on the ground.	Turn your legs to one side, then the other, while keeping your heels to the ground (movement of windscreen wipers).	Get back to the cross-legged position.

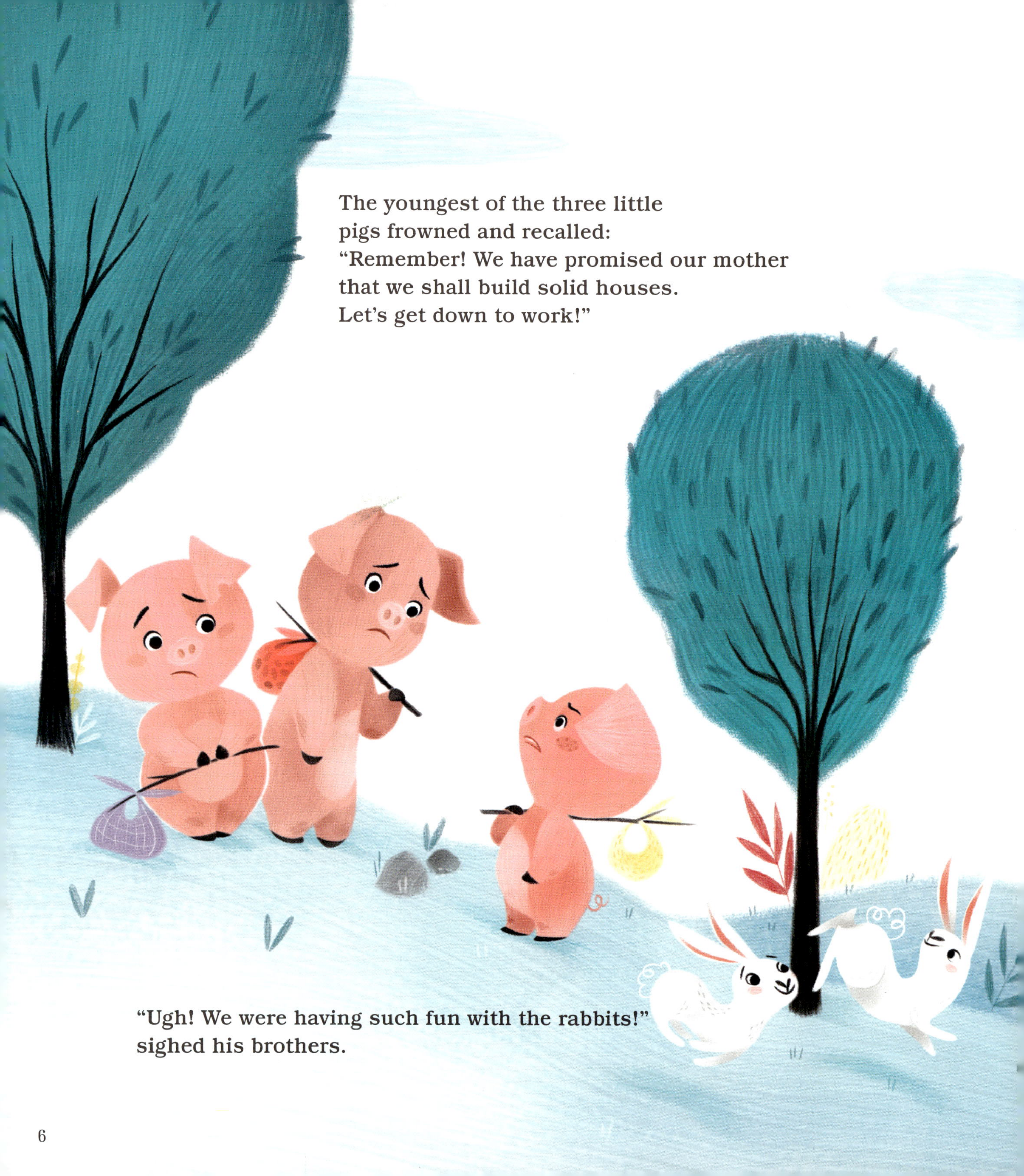

The youngest of the three little pigs frowned and recalled: "Remember! We have promised our mother that we shall build solid houses. Let's get down to work!"

"Ugh! We were having such fun with the rabbits!" sighed his brothers.

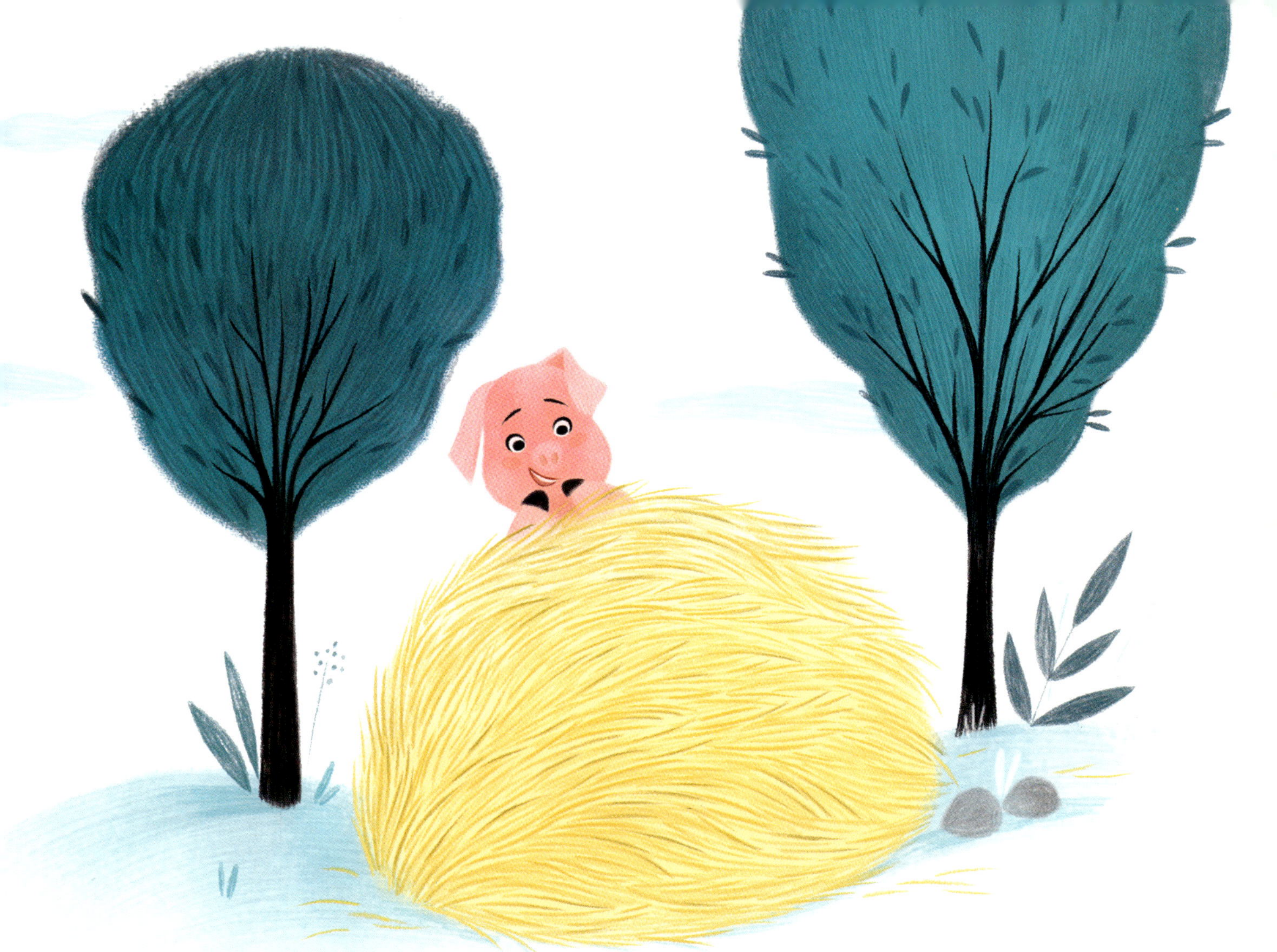

The first little pig spotted a round pile of straw
at the edge of the forest.
He thought: ‘This is exactly what I need!’

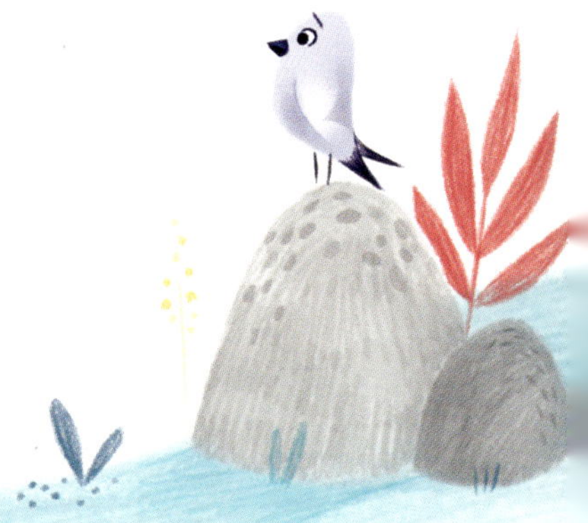

Immediately he dived into the huge pile of straw and disappeared in it. How nice it smelt!

"My house is ready!" he cried

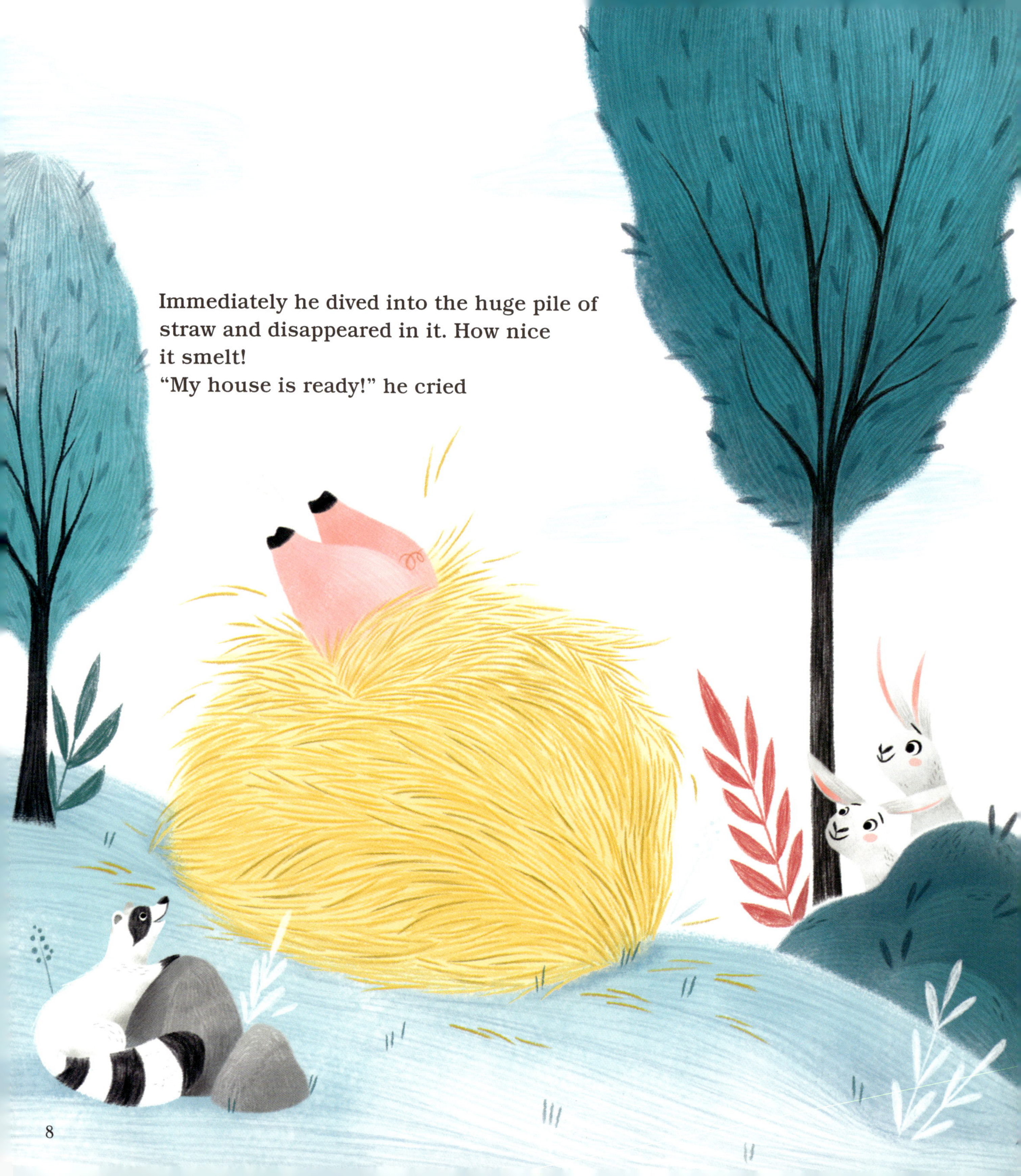

The second little pig observed the house of straw and declared:
"But it is not solid! Moreover, it doesn't even look like a house. There is no door for entering."

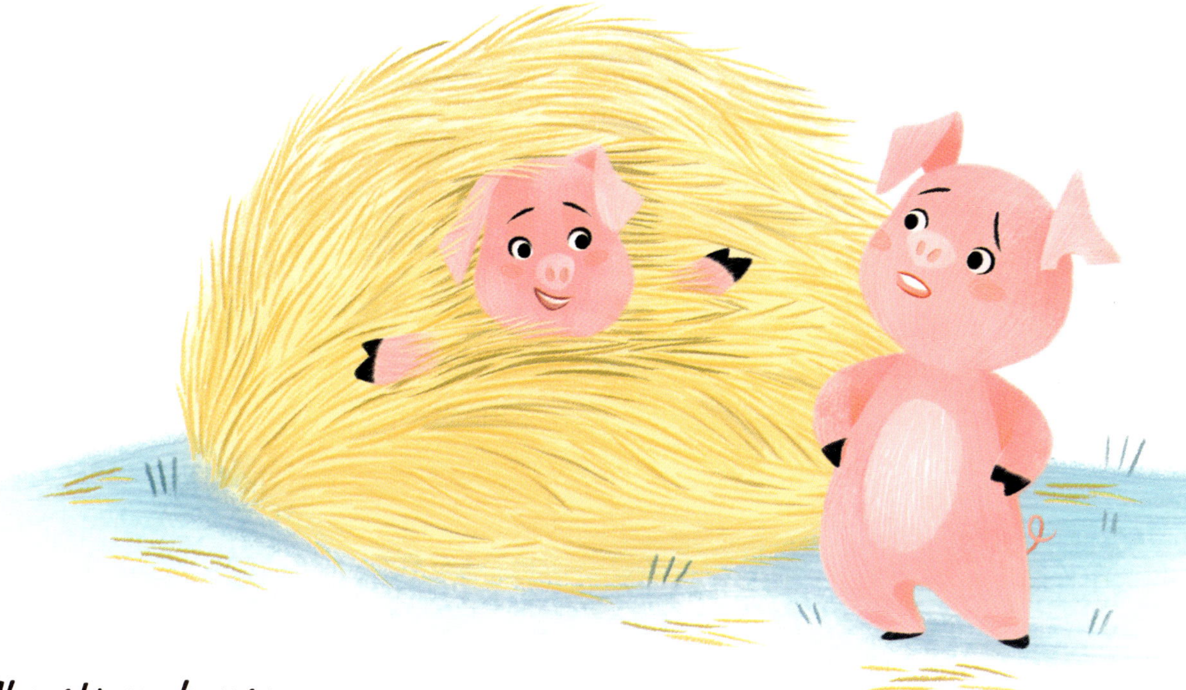

The straw house

You are as light as straw.

Benefit: This posture, to be done by two people, makes the abductors flexible.

4 times

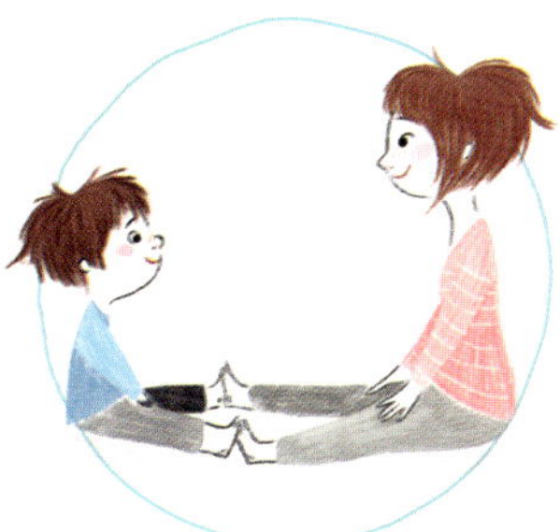

Sit facing each other. Place your legs in front of you, and hold them apart them like a pair of scissors.

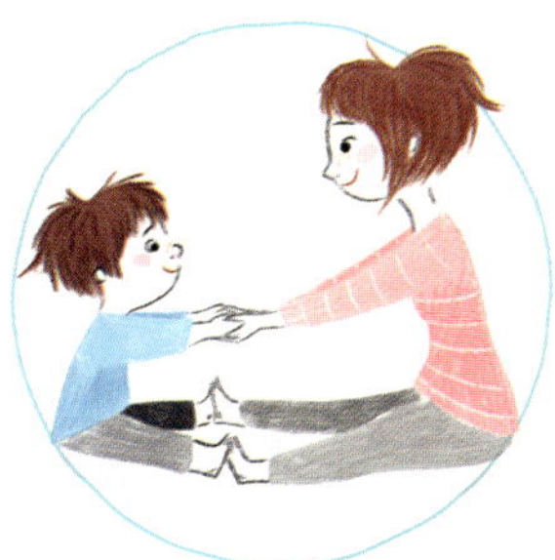

The soles of your feet must touch, and the adult must hold the child by his hands.

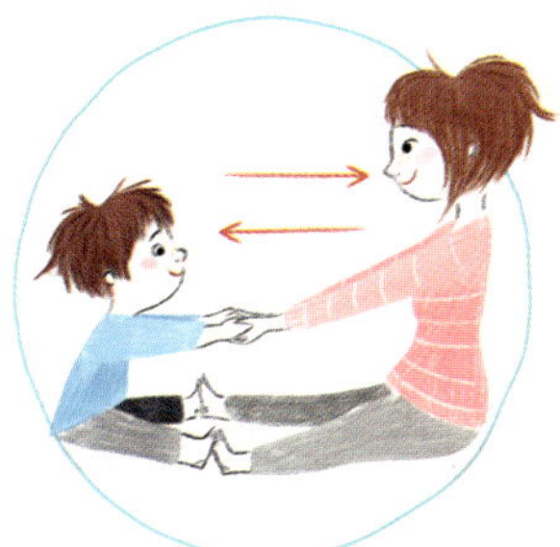

The child pulls the adult gently towards him. Then the movement is reversed.

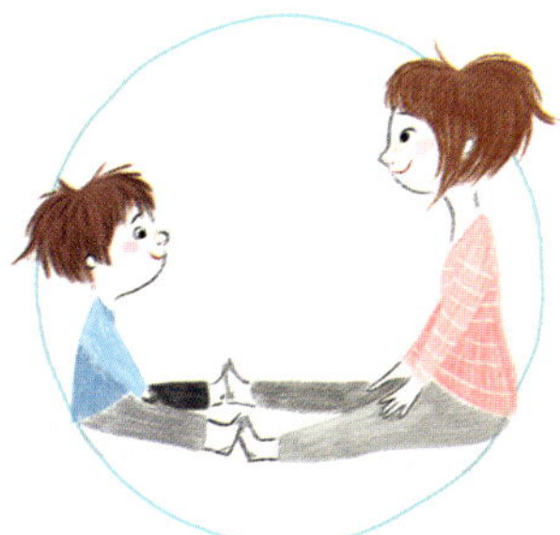

Let go of the hands gently and bring your legs back together.

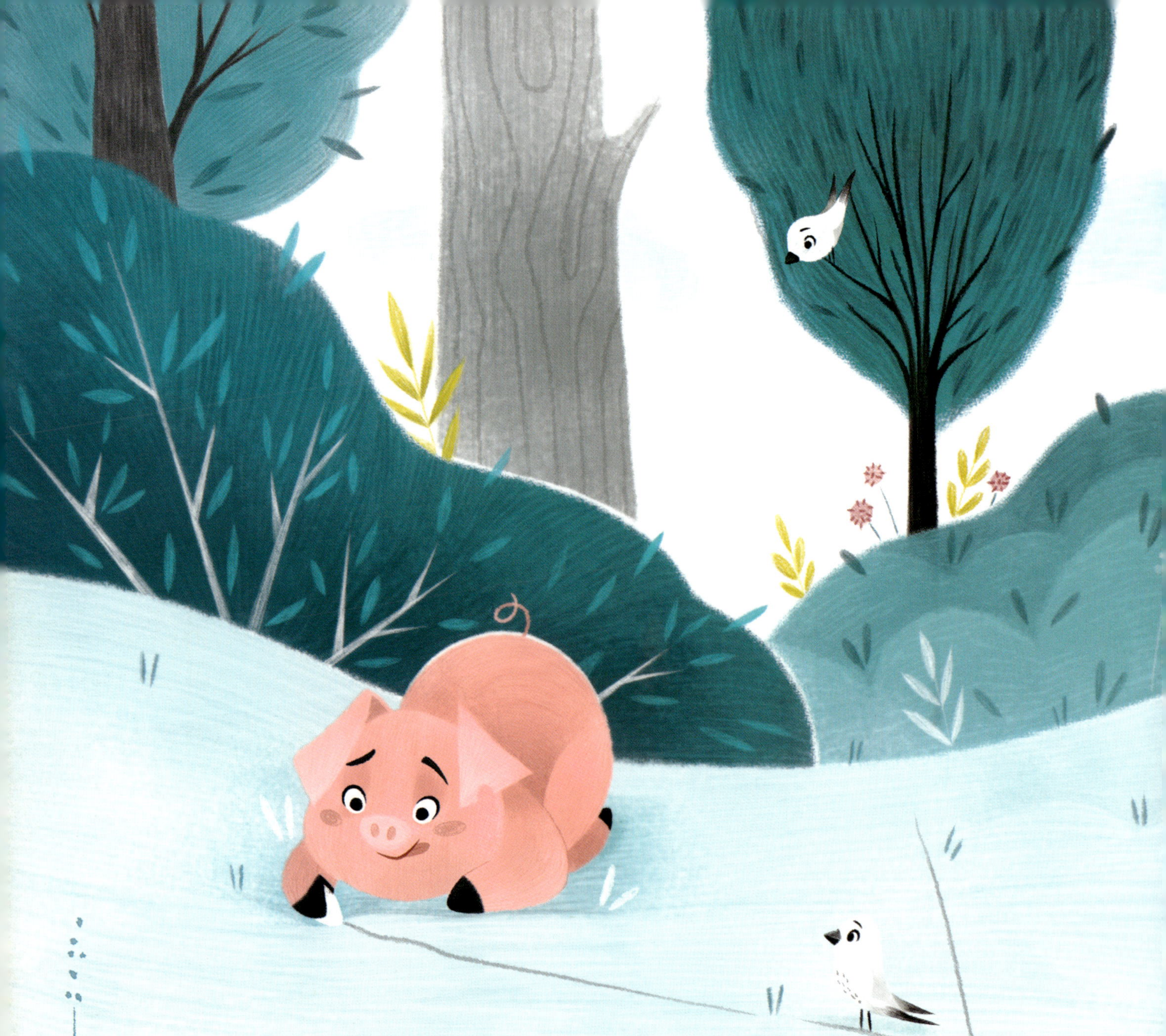

Then the second little pig looked around and thought of his future home. He drew a plan on the ground and remembered to draw a door and a window too.

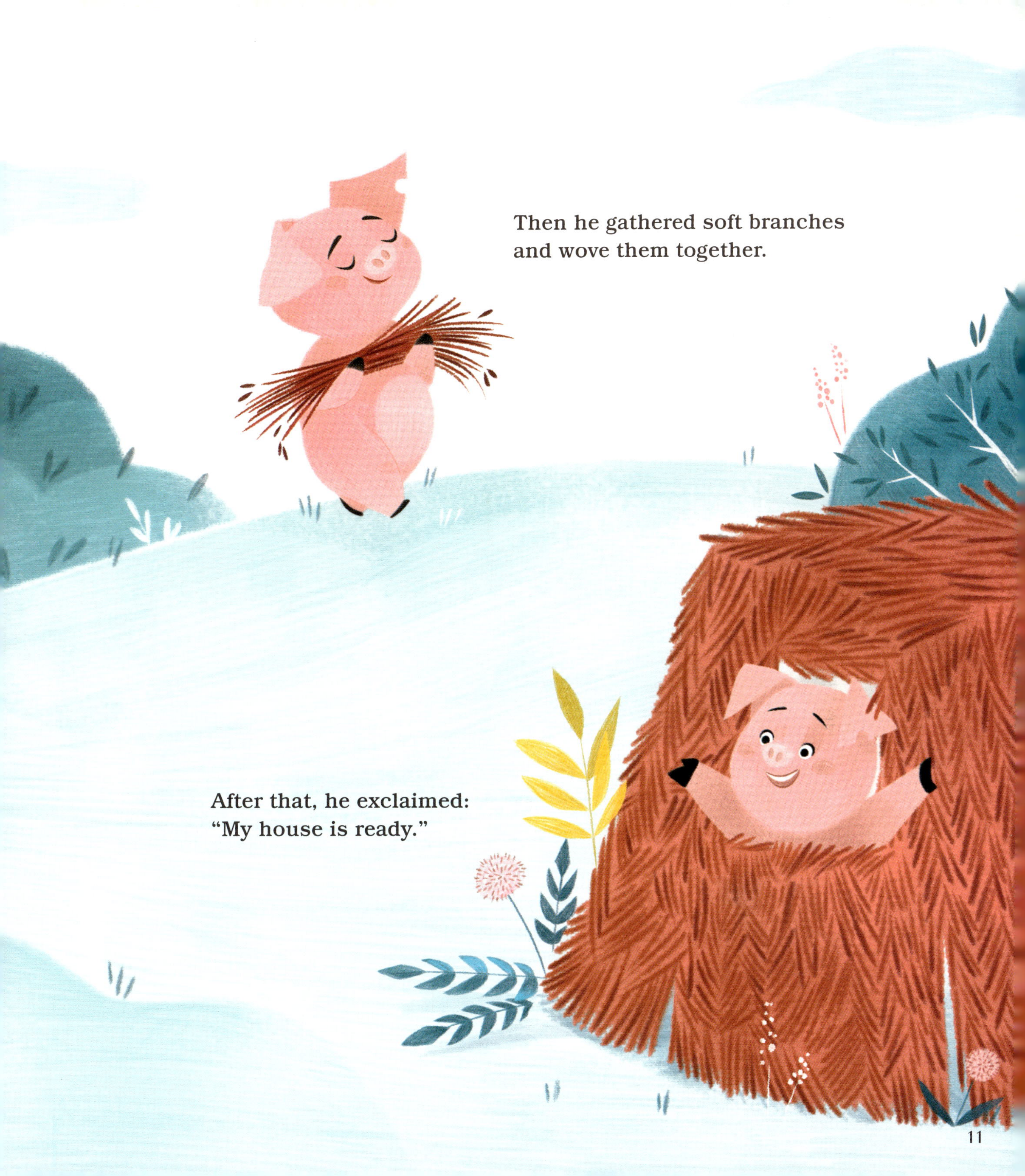

Then he gathered soft branches
and wove them together.

After that, he exclaimed:
"My house is ready."

This house looked like a huge wicker basket turned upside down.
The third little pig looked at it and started sulking. He shook his head:
“No, no, my brothers, these houses are just not solid enough.”

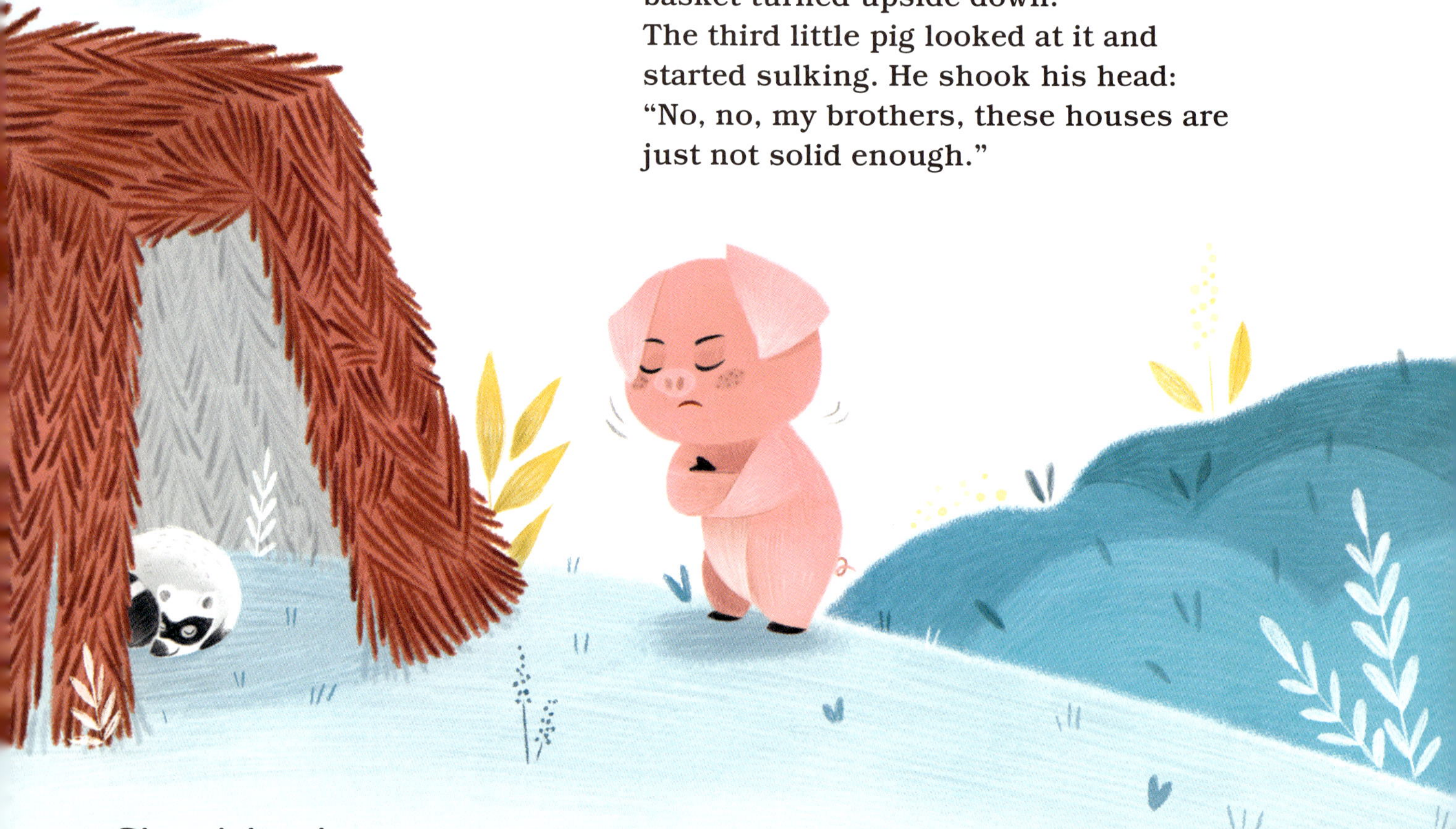

The wicker house

You are as flexible as wicker.

Benefit: This posture helps make the posterior muscle chain flexible.

5 breaths

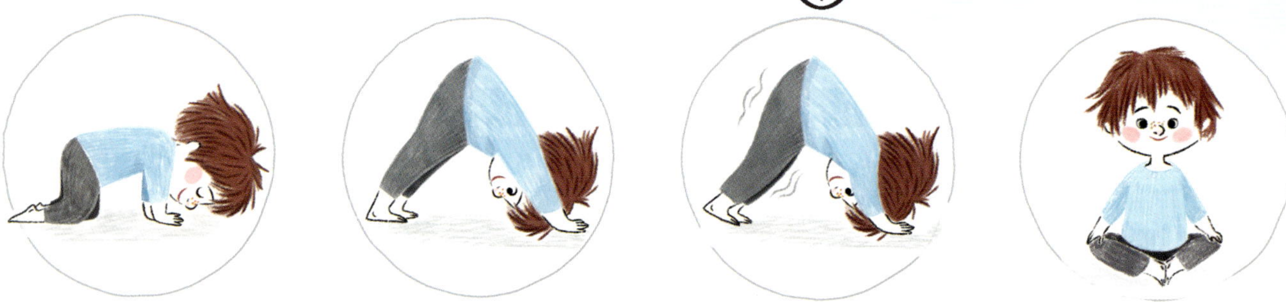

Get down on all fours.

Lift the pelvis while pushing the ground with your hands. Your body forms a toboggan.

Enjoy moving the toboggan gently first with your legs, then with your hands.

Sit down on your heels. Thereafter, sit cross-legged.

“Don’t be difficult! It’s quite solid this way. Come and play with us, instead,” exclaimed the brothers.

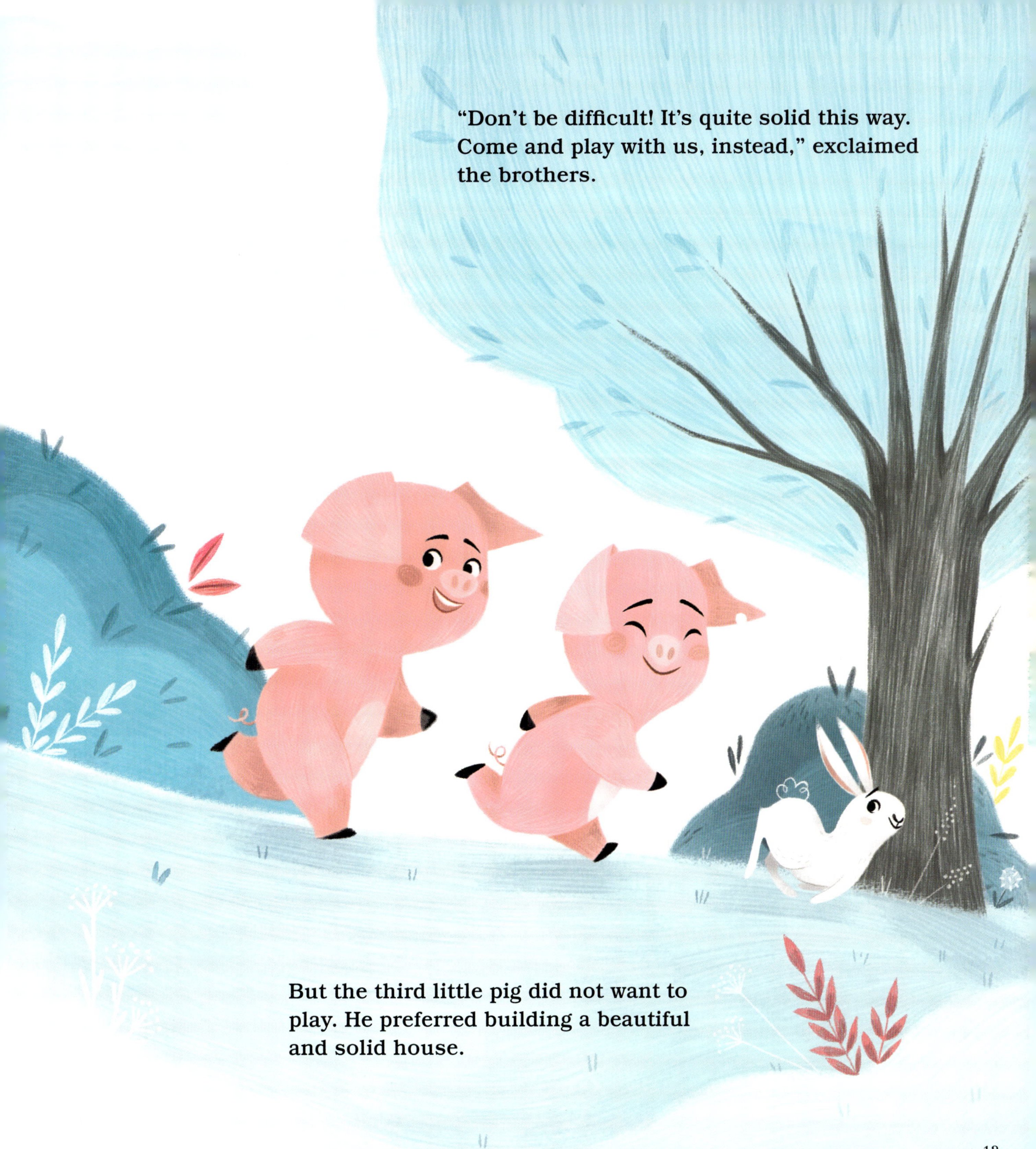

But the third little pig did not want to play. He preferred building a beautiful and solid house.

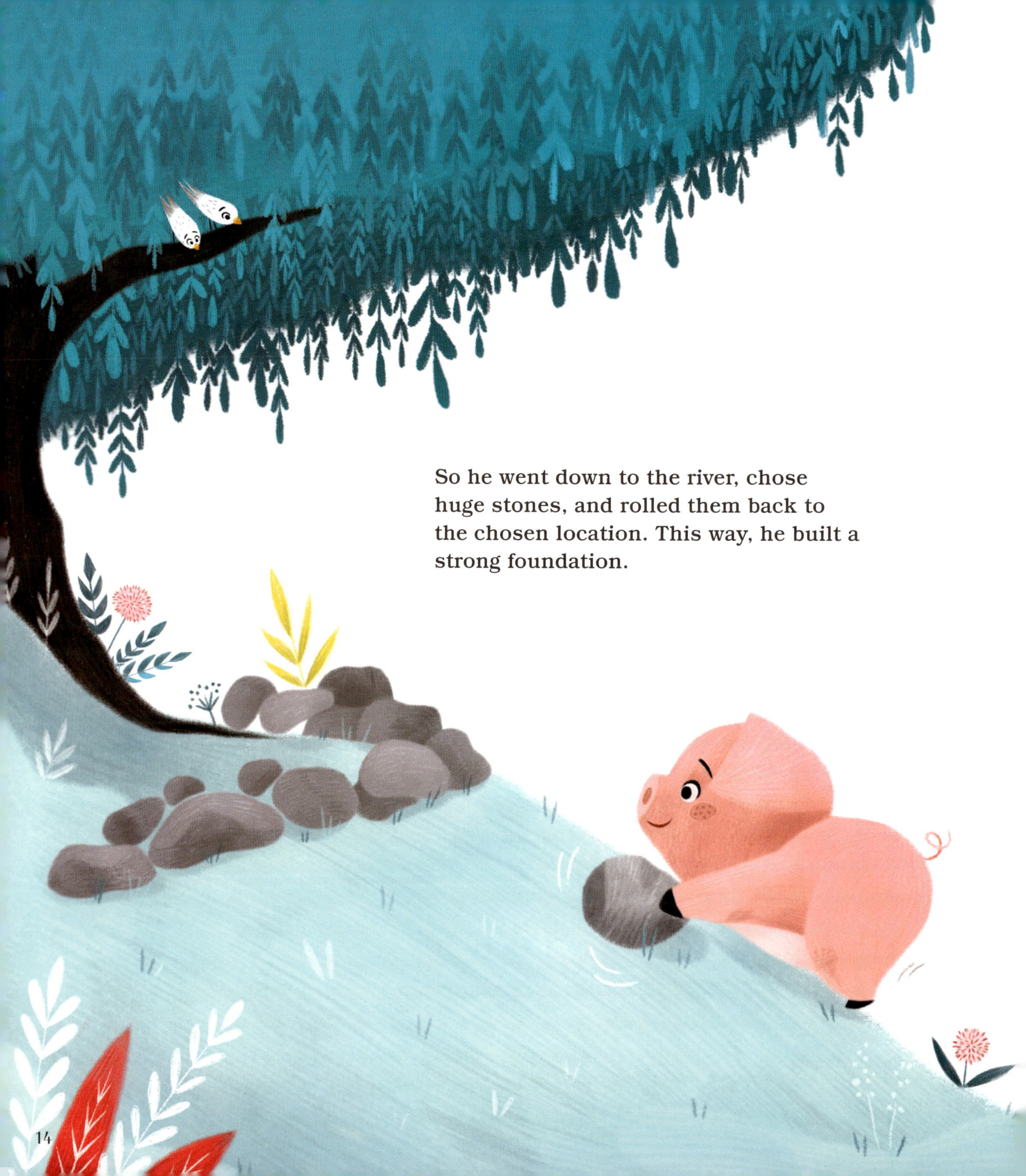

So he went down to the river, chose huge stones, and rolled them back to the chosen location. This way, he built a strong foundation.

At the waterfront, he also discovered a place where the soil was humid and soft. Clay! What fun to be rolling in it!

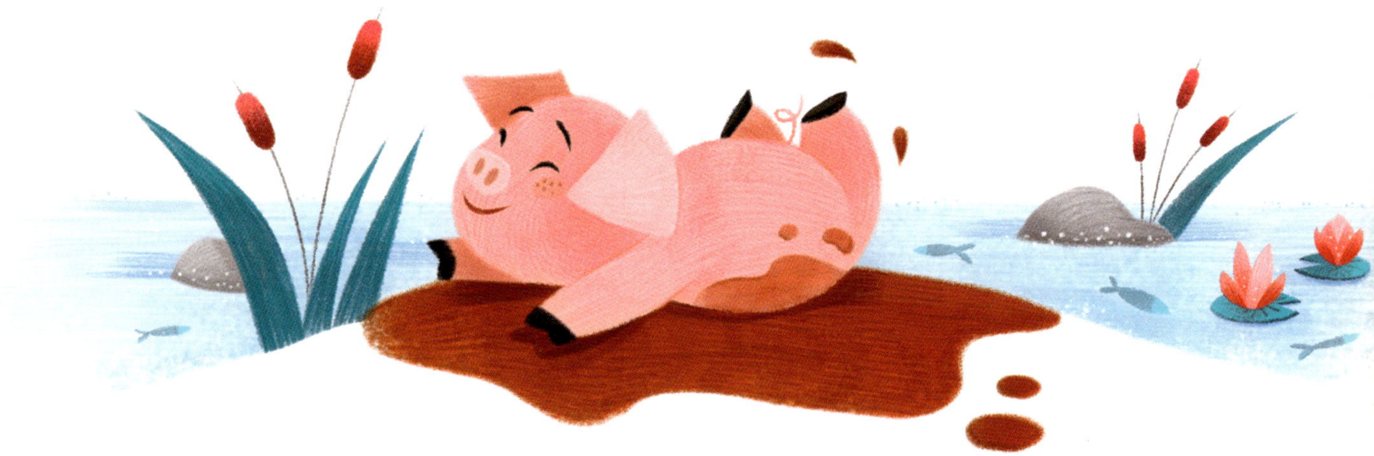

'Impossible to stay away! Oink-oink, it is refreshing and has made my skin so soft.'

The roll

Like the little pig, roll in the mud.

Benefit: This posture provides a self-massage of the spine.

4 times

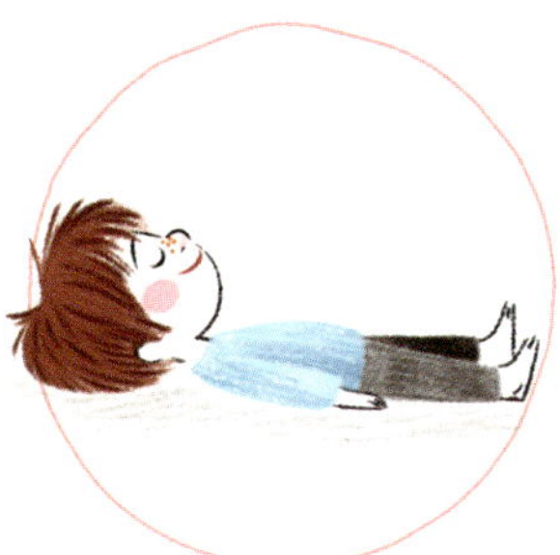

Lie down, with your back gently on the ground.

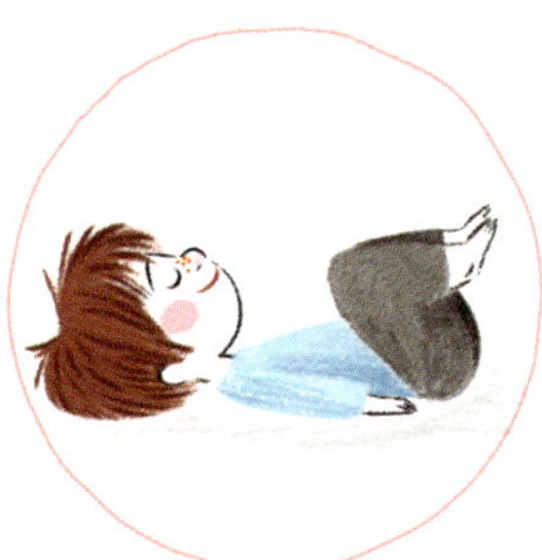

Fold your legs. Hold your knees above your chest.

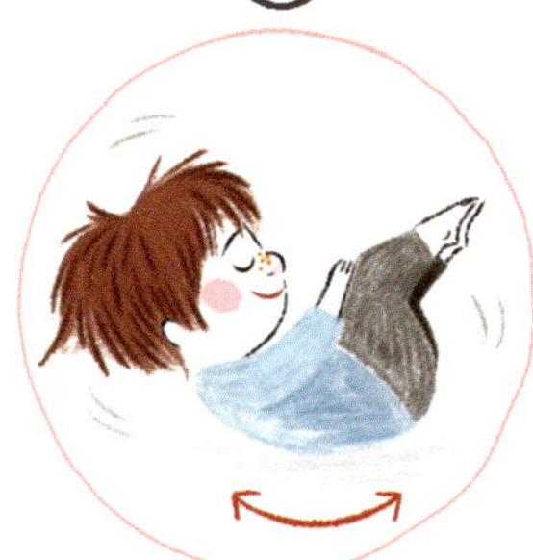

Hug your knees. Bend the spine and take in the chin. Rock gently from back to front.

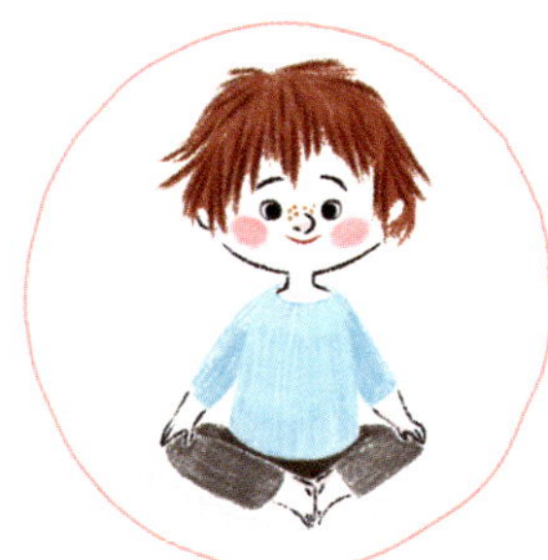

Get back to sitting cross-legged.

He set about coating the walls of the house with clay, while swallows plugged the holes with some feathers and strands of herbs. Some work that was!

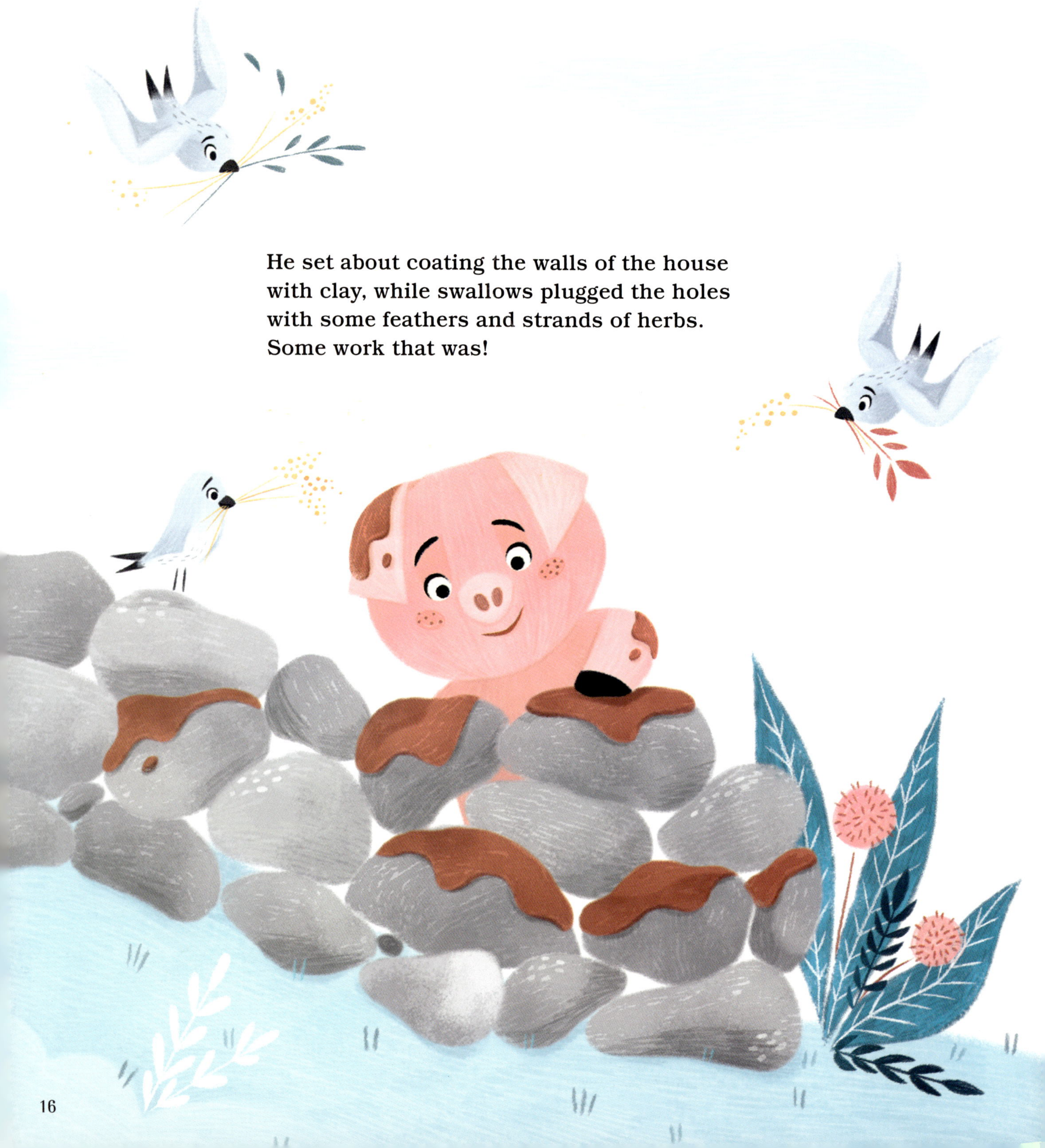

'That trunk shall make a fine beam to support the roof.'
He lifted it on his back. Gosh, was it heavy!

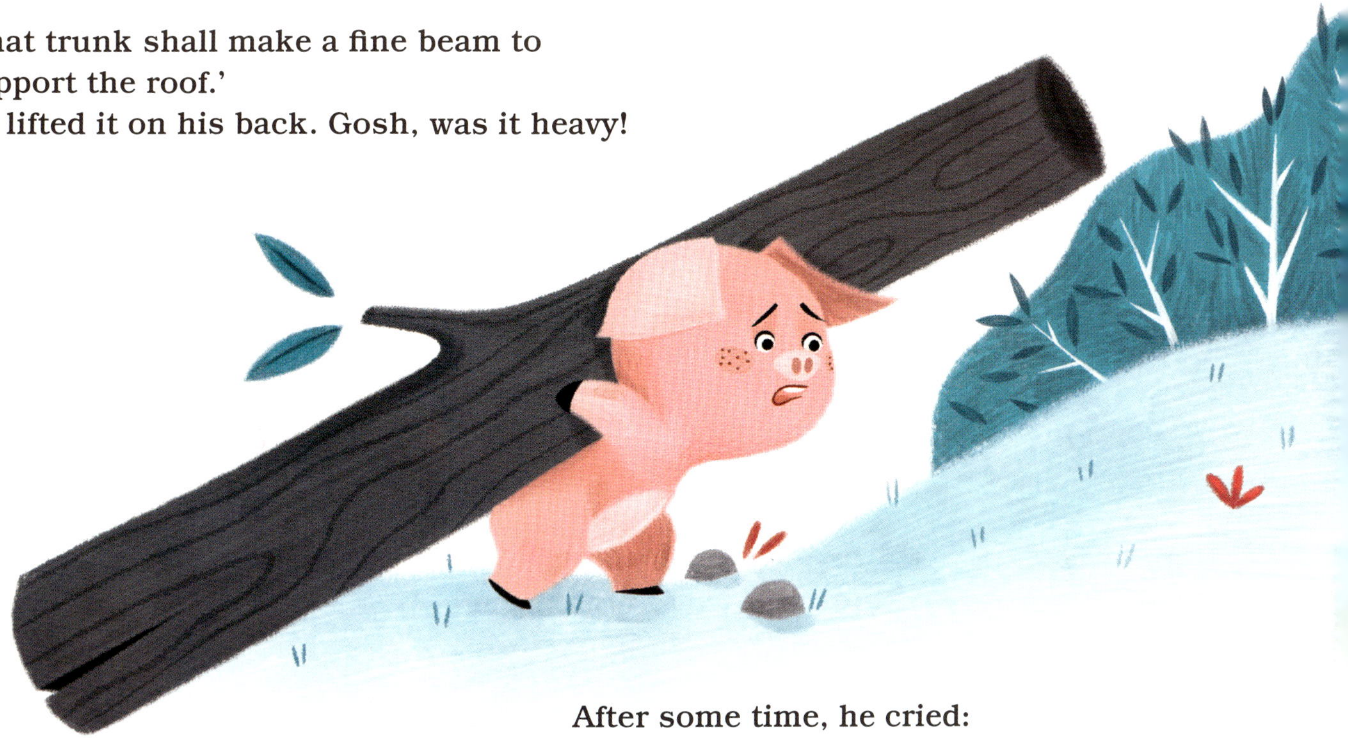

After some time, he cried:
"My house is ready!"
Everything was in place, including a chimney.

The chimney

With two people, make a fine chimney.
Benefit: This posture helps become aware of the spine.

5 breaths

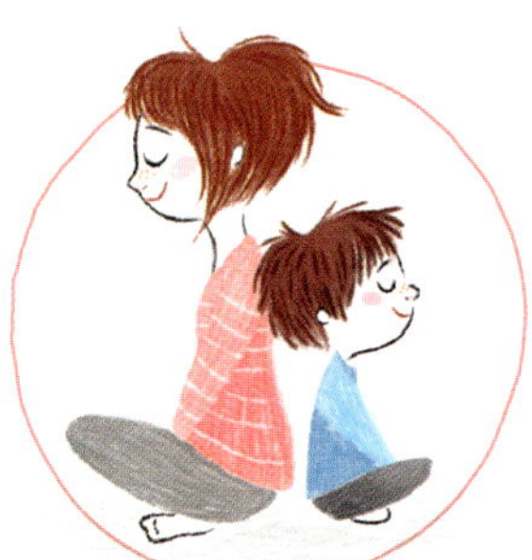

Sit cross-legged, back-to-back.

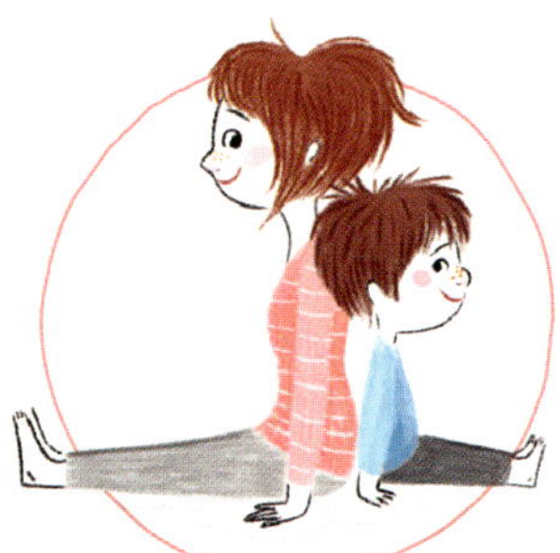

Join your legs and stretch them in front of you. Keep your arms on each side of the torso, and push the ground with your hands.

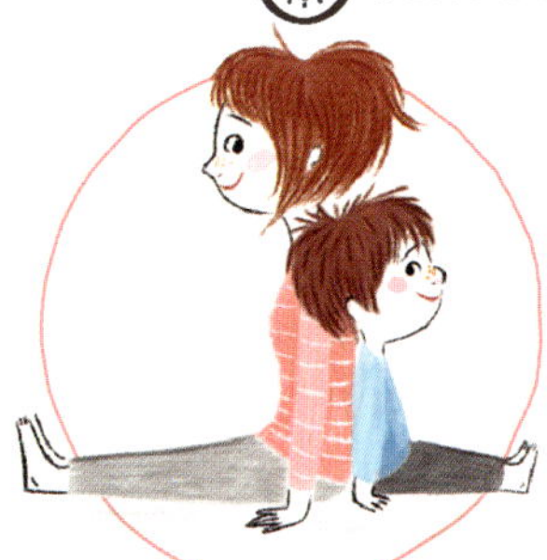

Adjust the posture so that the torsos form a rectangle.

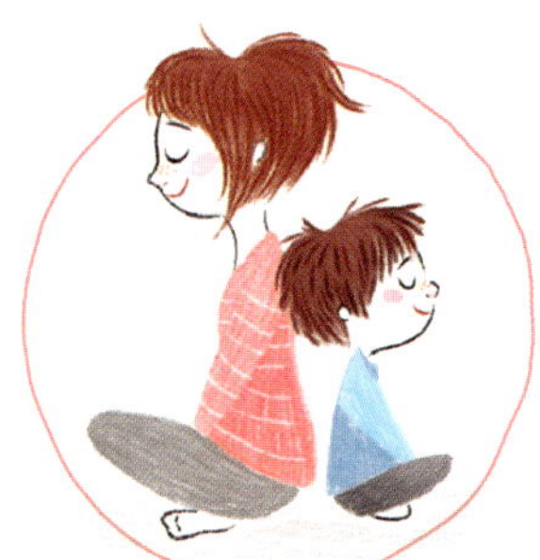

Undo the posture and get back to sitting cross-legged.

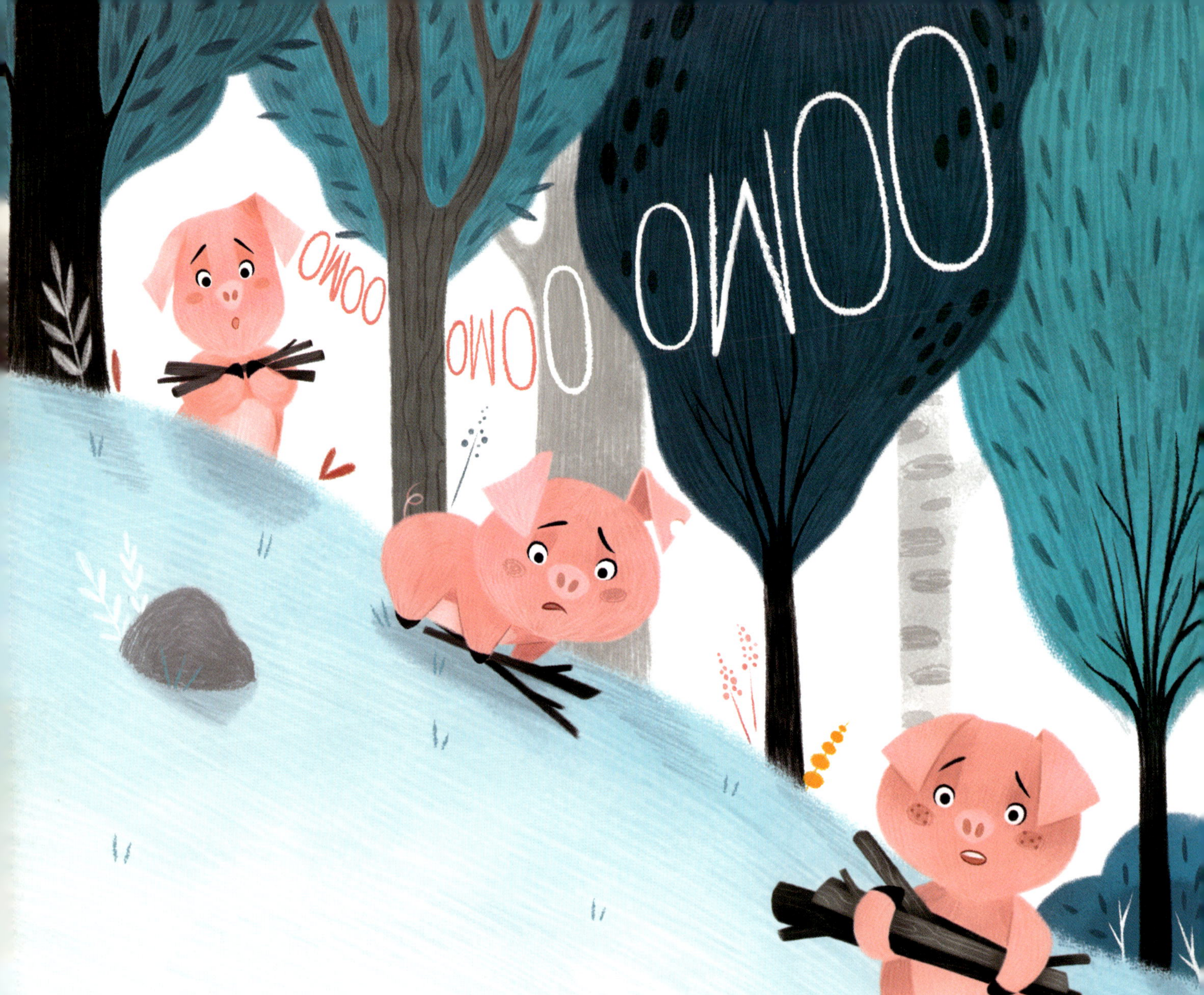

That evening, while the three little pigs were gathering wood to cook their meal, in the distance, they heard a worrying cry:
"Owoo, owoo, owoo..."
"It is the wolf! Hurry everybody, get inside!"

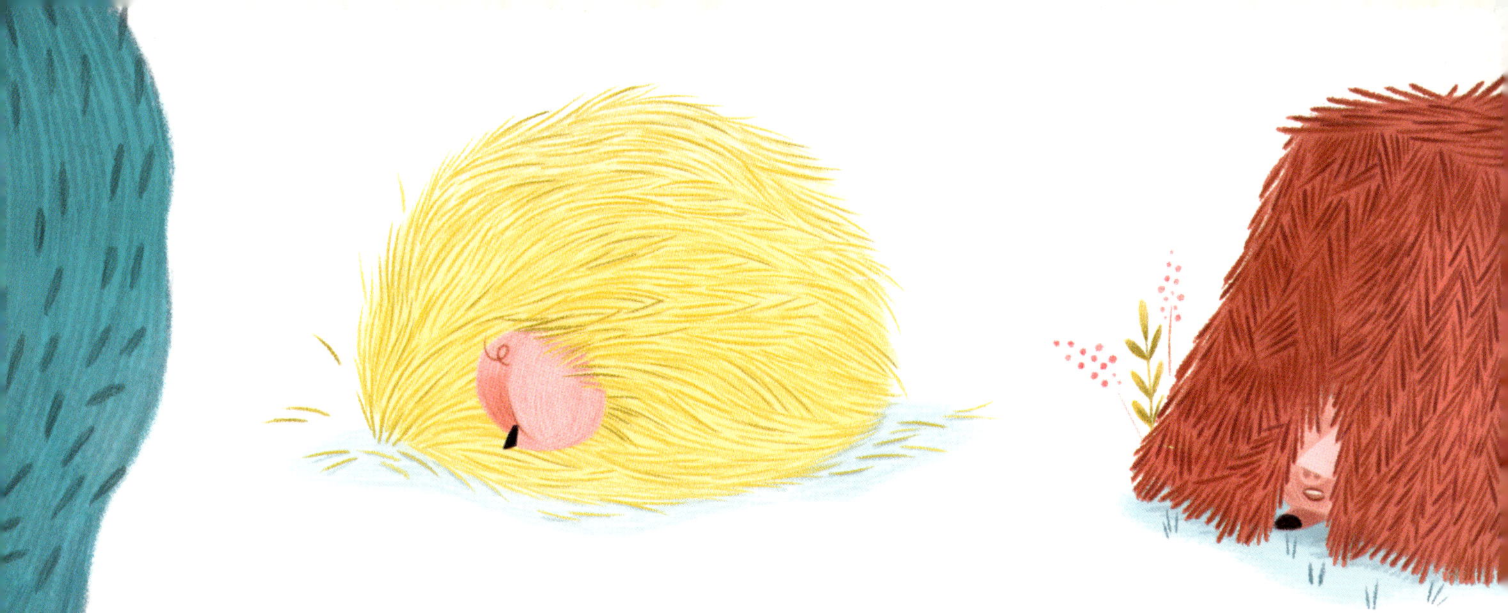

The first little pig dived into his pile of straw.
The second little pig ran into his wicker hut.
The third little pig returned to his house, slammed shut the windows, and locked the door with the key.

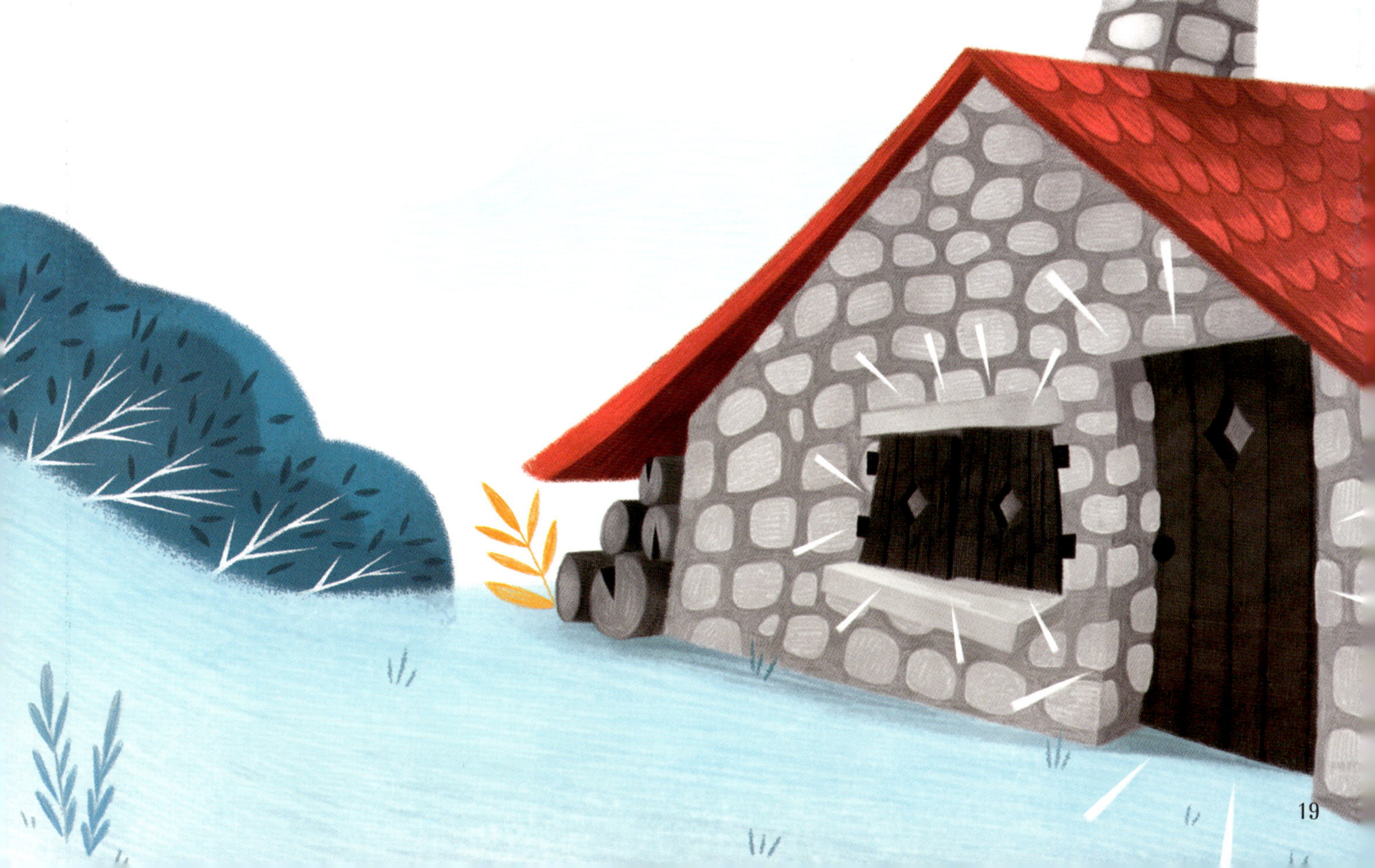

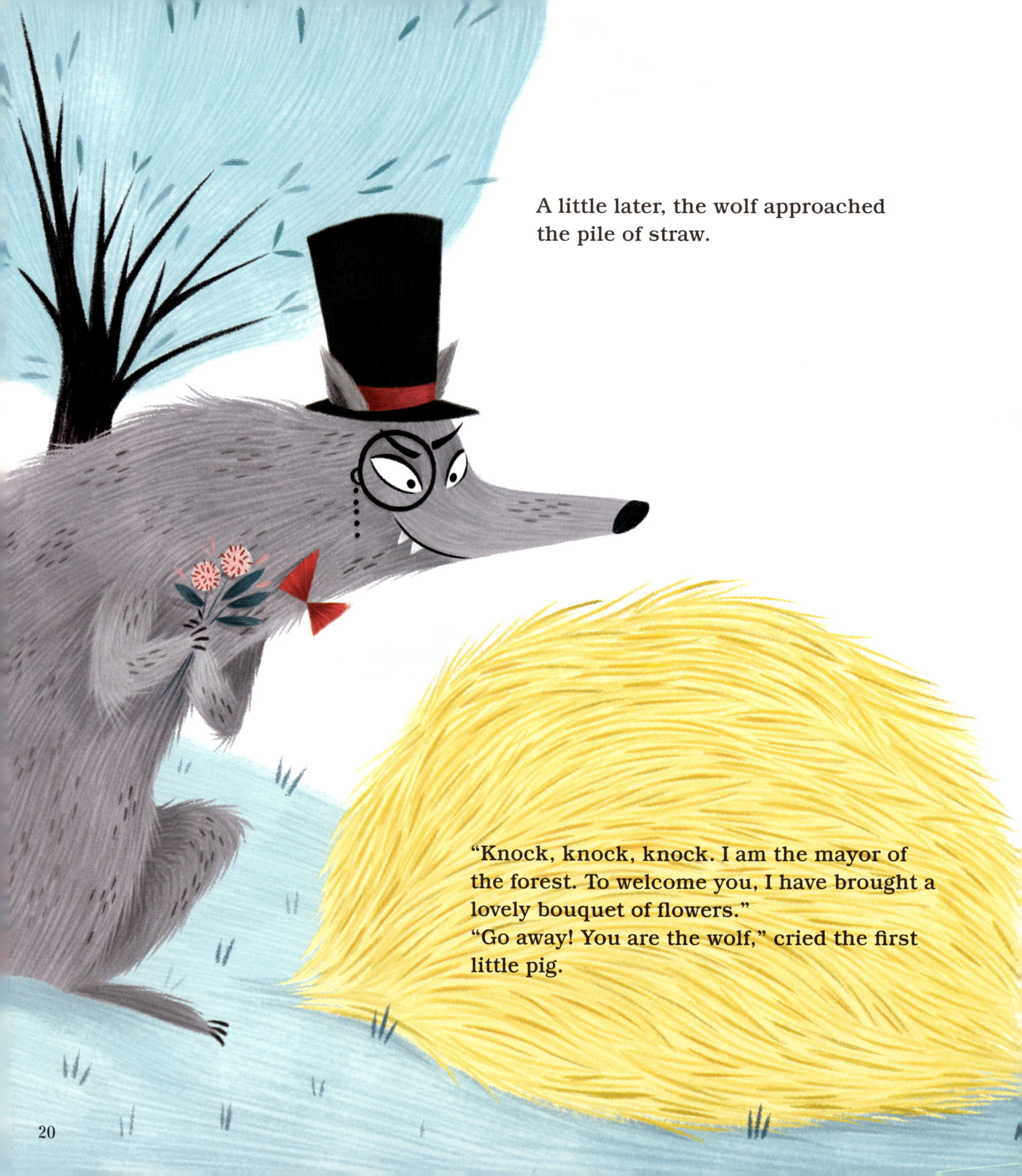

A little later, the wolf approached the pile of straw.

“Knock, knock, knock. I am the mayor of the forest. To welcome you, I have brought a lovely bouquet of flowers.”

“Go away! You are the wolf,” cried the first little pig.

“Well! I shall blow and I shall spit so hard that your house shall fly away!”

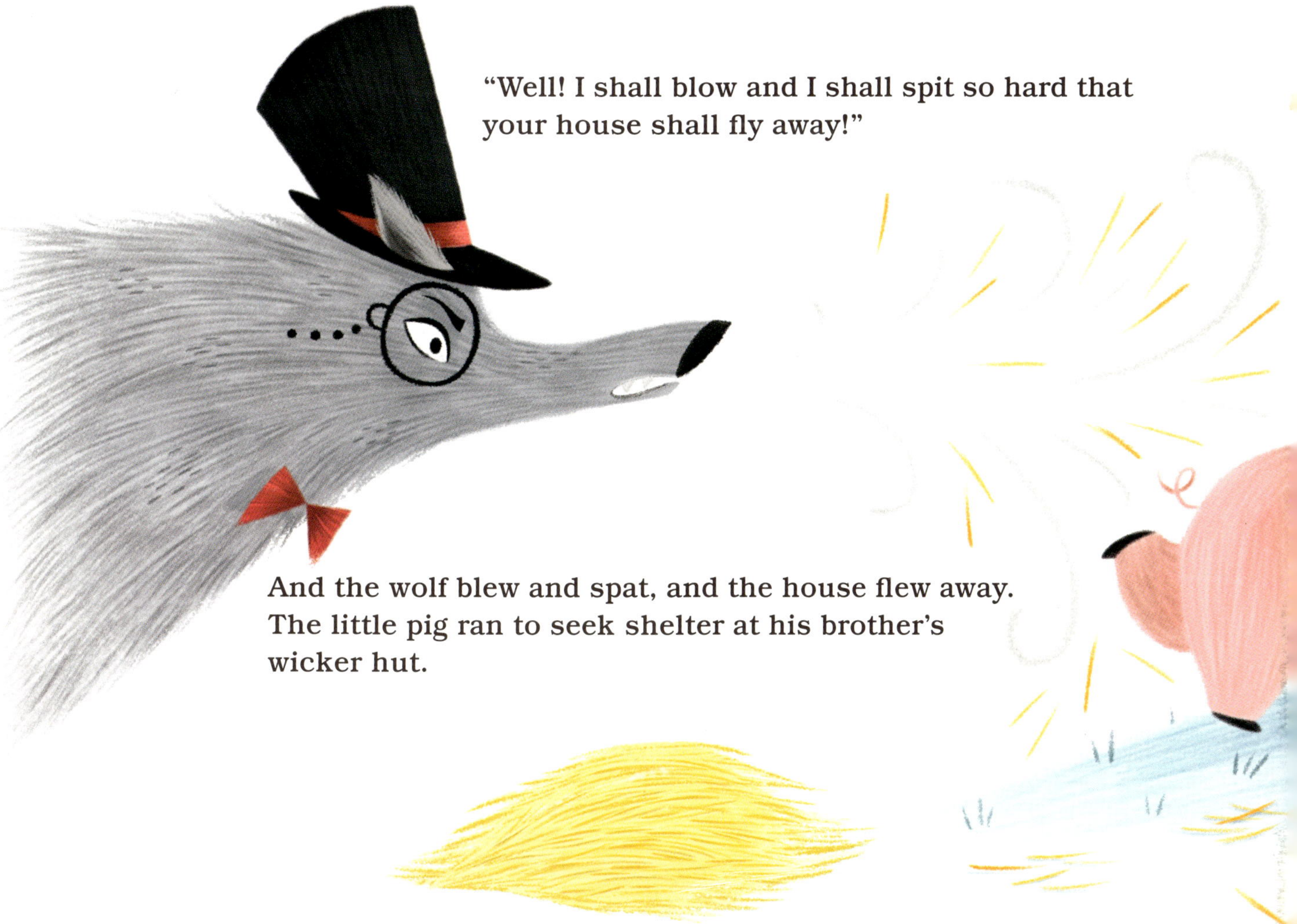

And the wolf blew and spat, and the house flew away. The little pig ran to seek shelter at his brother’s wicker hut.

The wolf blowing

Blow hard like the wolf!

Benefits: This posture gets rid of tension and opens up the mind to imagination.

3 times

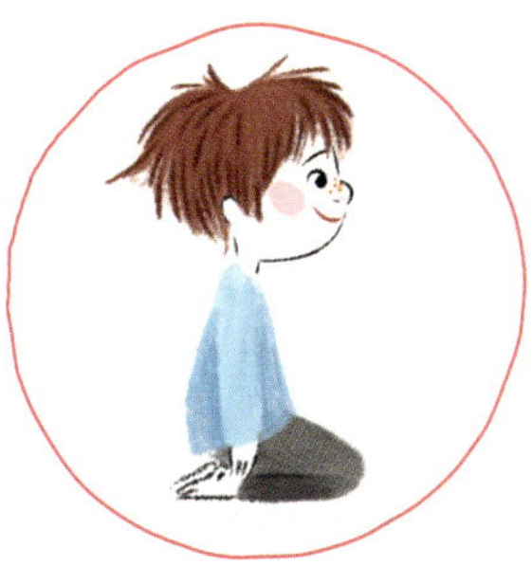

Sit on your heels, with your hands by the side of your body.

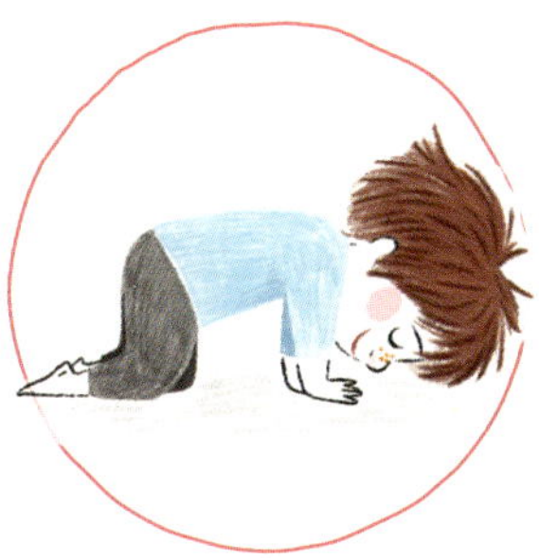

Place your hands on the ground, so you are on all fours.

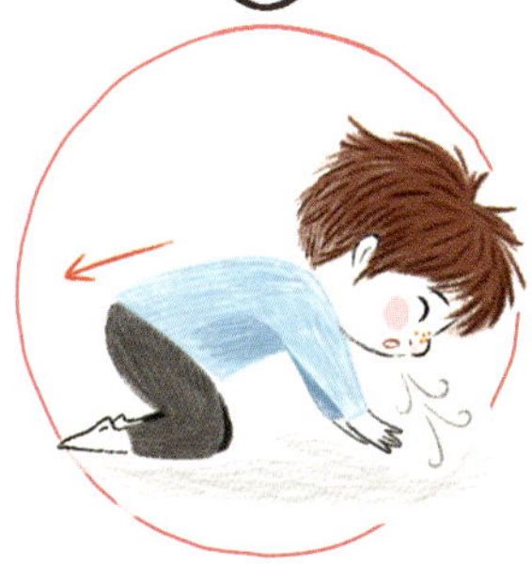

Move your pelvis back towards the heels. Take a deep breath through the nose and blow hard from the mouth.

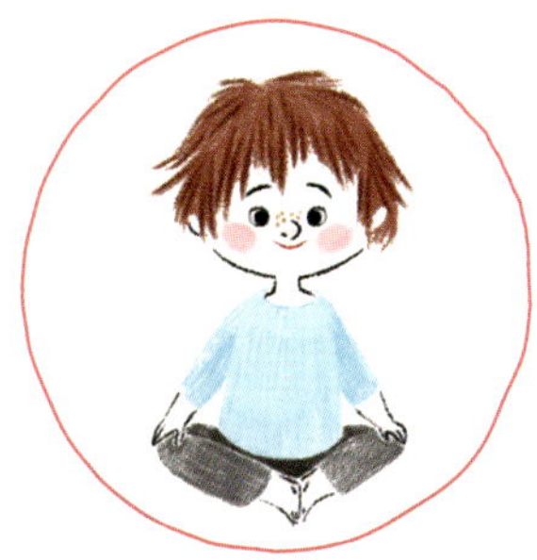

Undo the posture and sit on your heels, then get back to sitting cross-legged.

The wolf made haste to arrive.
"Knock, knock, knock. I am the doctor of the forest. Have you thought of getting yourself vaccinated?"
"Go away! You are the wolf," cried the second little pig.

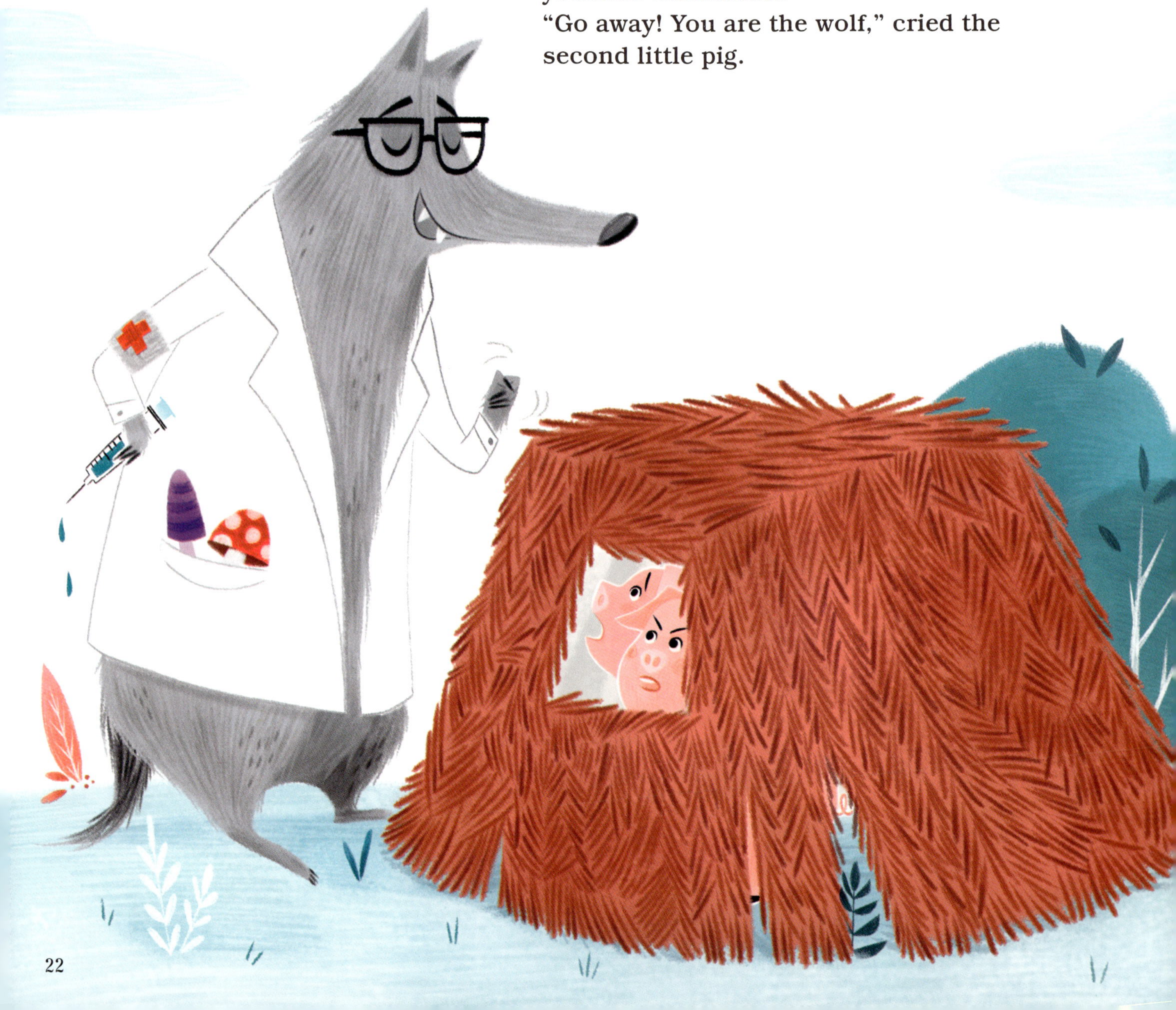

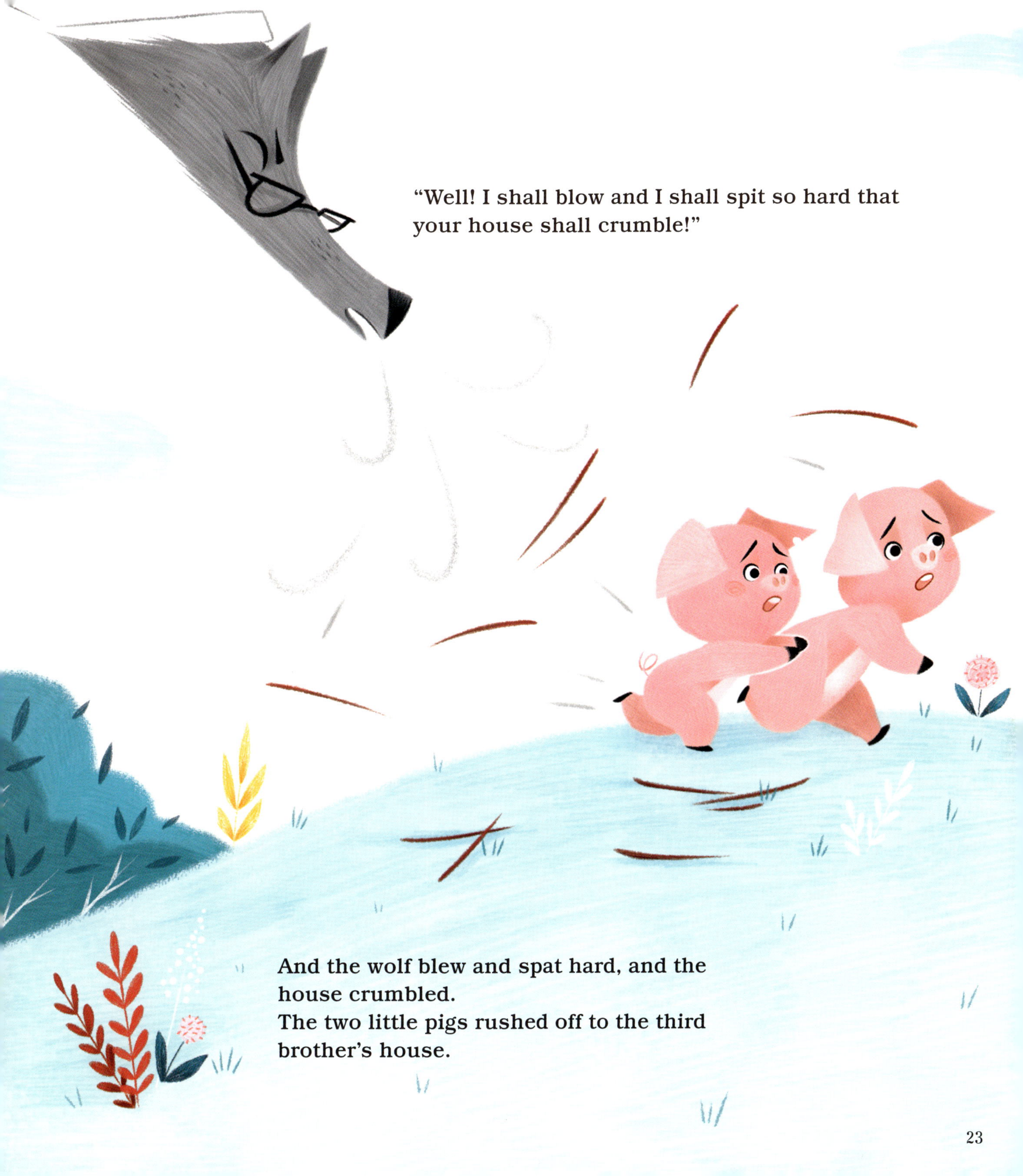

"Well! I shall blow and I shall spit so hard that your house shall crumble!"

And the wolf blew and spat hard, and the house crumbled.
The two little pigs rushed off to the third brother's house.

A short while later, the wolf appeared in front of the stone house.
"Knock, knock, knock. I am the cook of the forest. In the menu is fern gratin. Care for a bite?"
"Go away! You are the wolf," cried the third little pig.

"You can disguise yourself all you want but we recognise you. By the hair of my chin, you shall not enter my house."

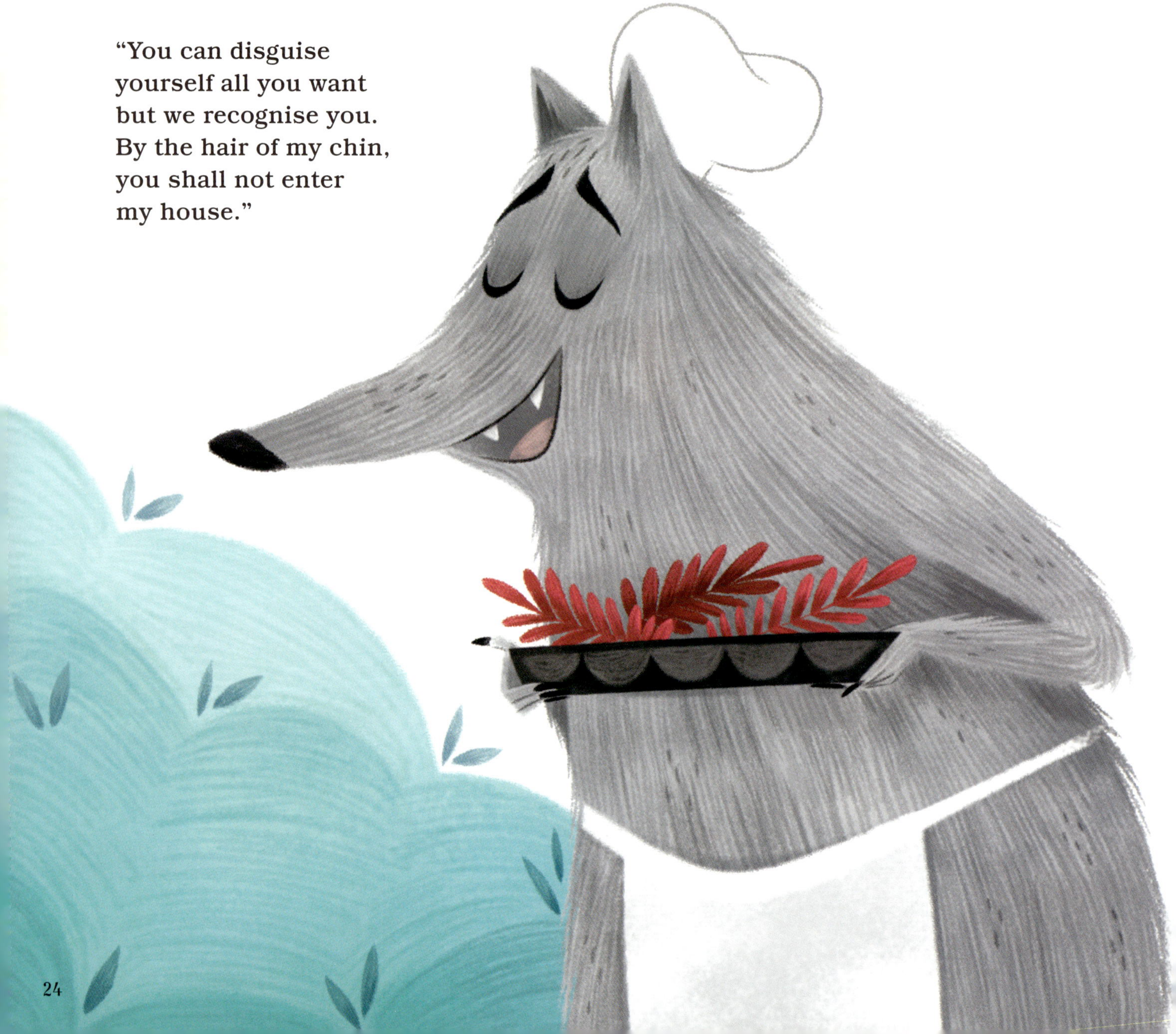

The wolf flew into a rage and yelled:
"I shall blow and I shall spit so hard that your house shall collapse!"

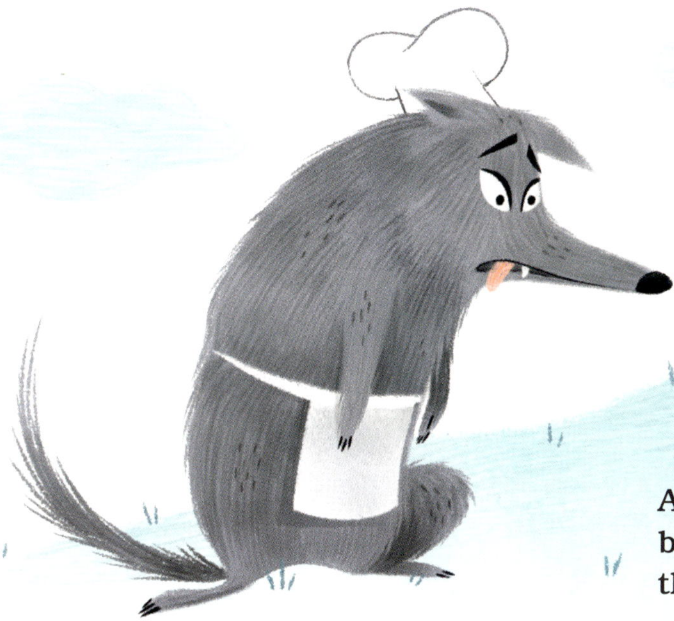

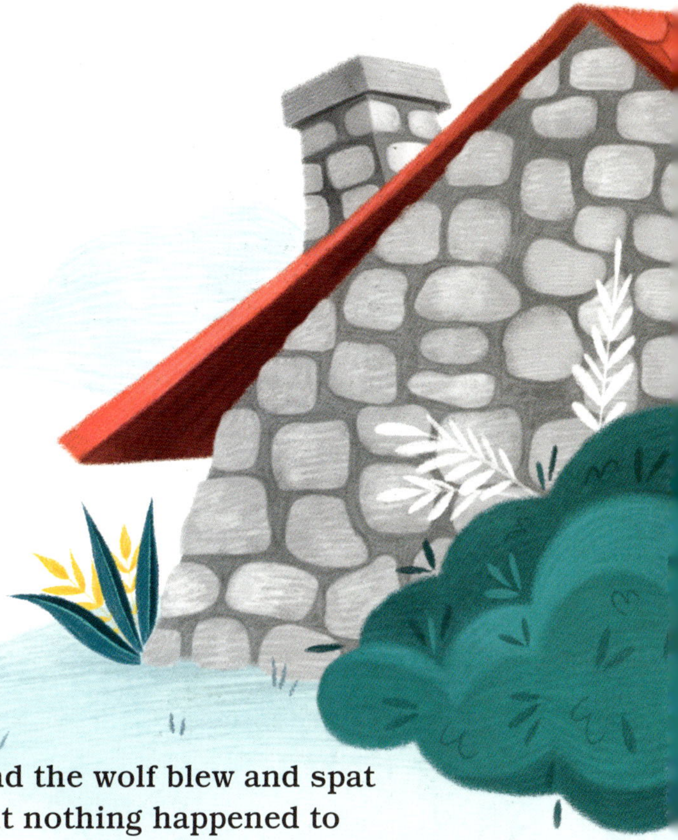

And the wolf blew and spat but nothing happened to the house.

The stone house

You are as strong as the stone.

Benefits: This posture is good for strength and stability.

5 breaths

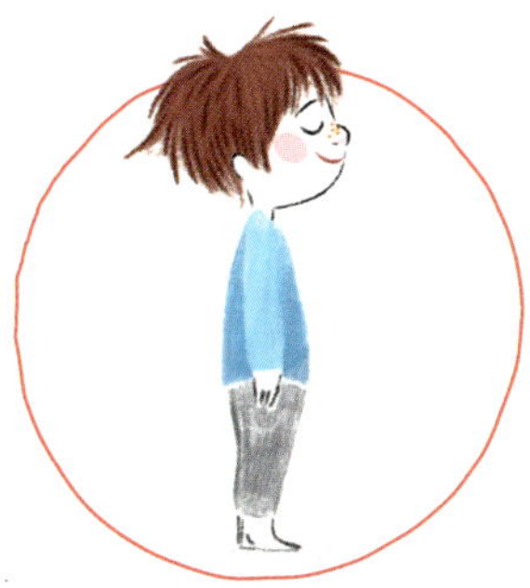

Stand so that your body is in a fine straight line.

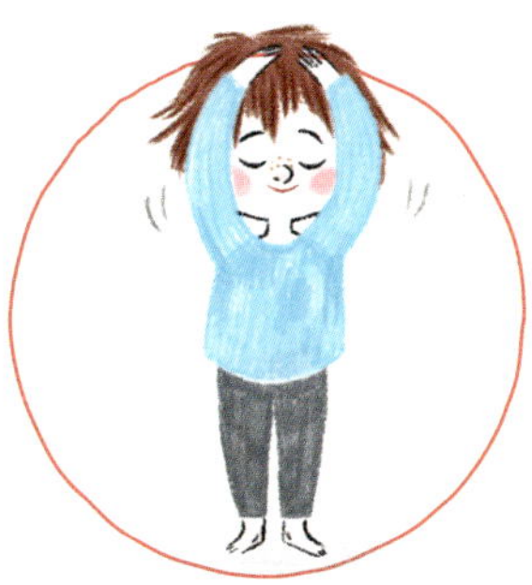

Lift your hands from the front and join the palms above your head.

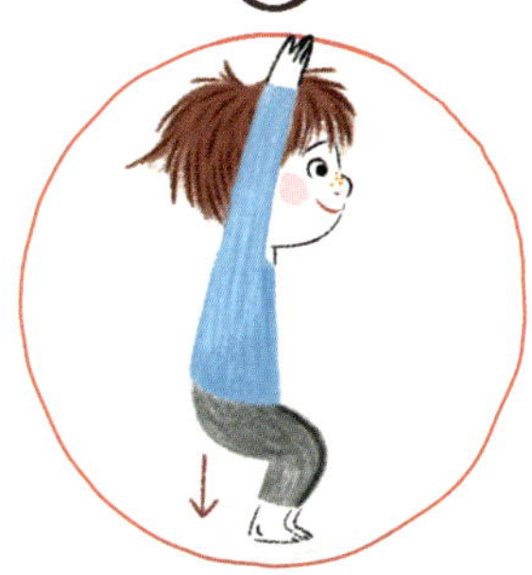

Flex your knees as though you are going to sit on a chair. Keep your back straight. Dig your heels into the ground.

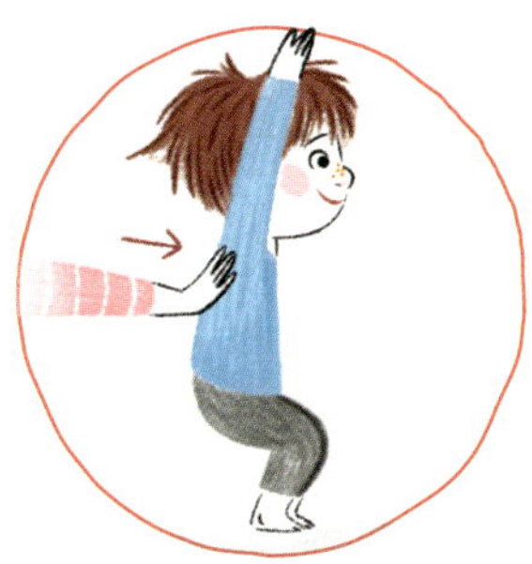

The adult tests the solidness of the house by gently placing the hands against the back of the child. Then the child gets back to the initial posture and relaxes his body.

So the wolf went around the house, lifted his head and hit upon an idea: "I shall climb up the roof and enter through the chimney to eat up the three little pigs, well grilled."

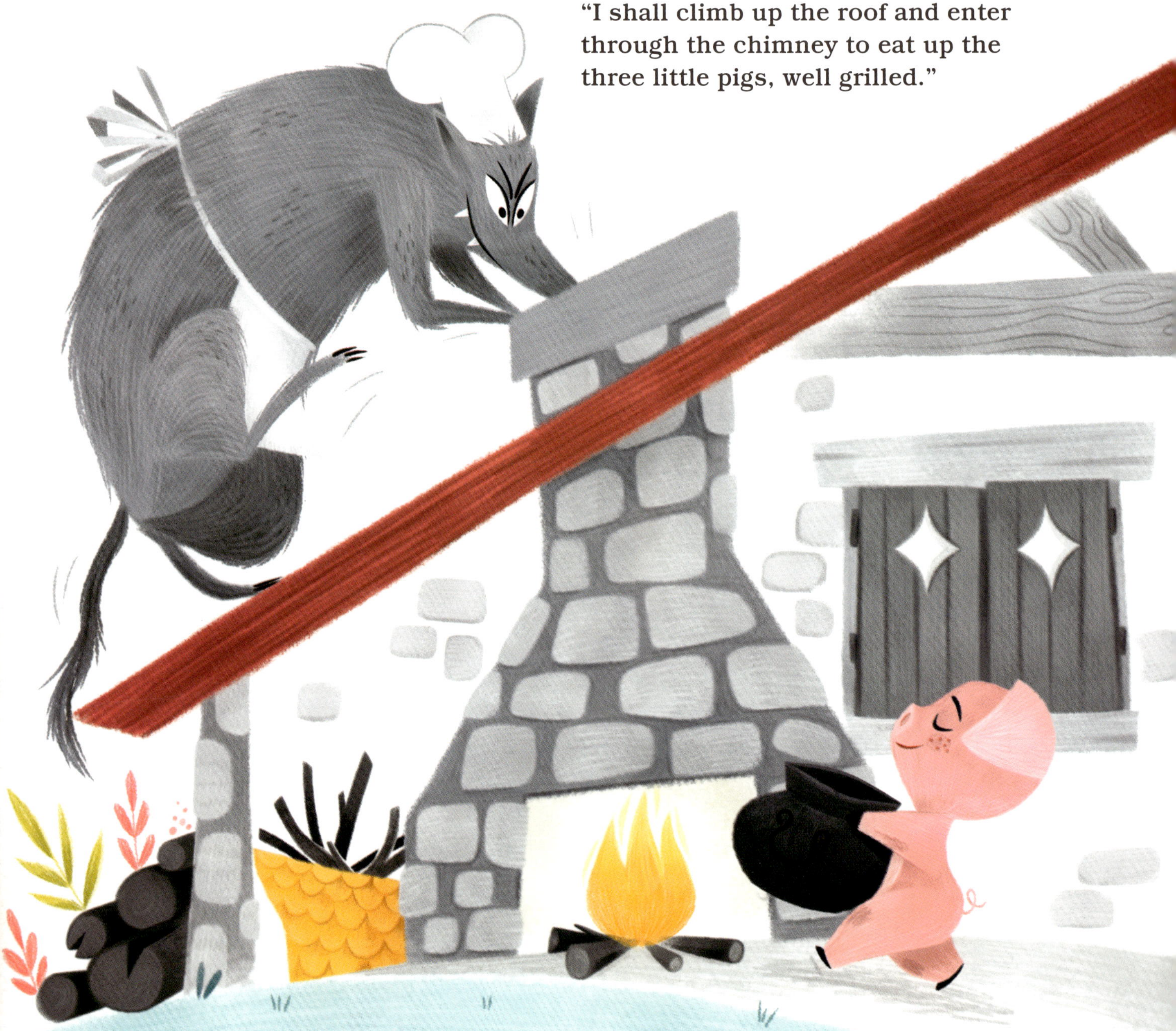

But the third little pig was clever. He placed a huge pot on the fire and the wolf fell into the boiling water.

“Ouch, ouch ouch,” screamed the wolf as he ran out of the door with his backside smoking.

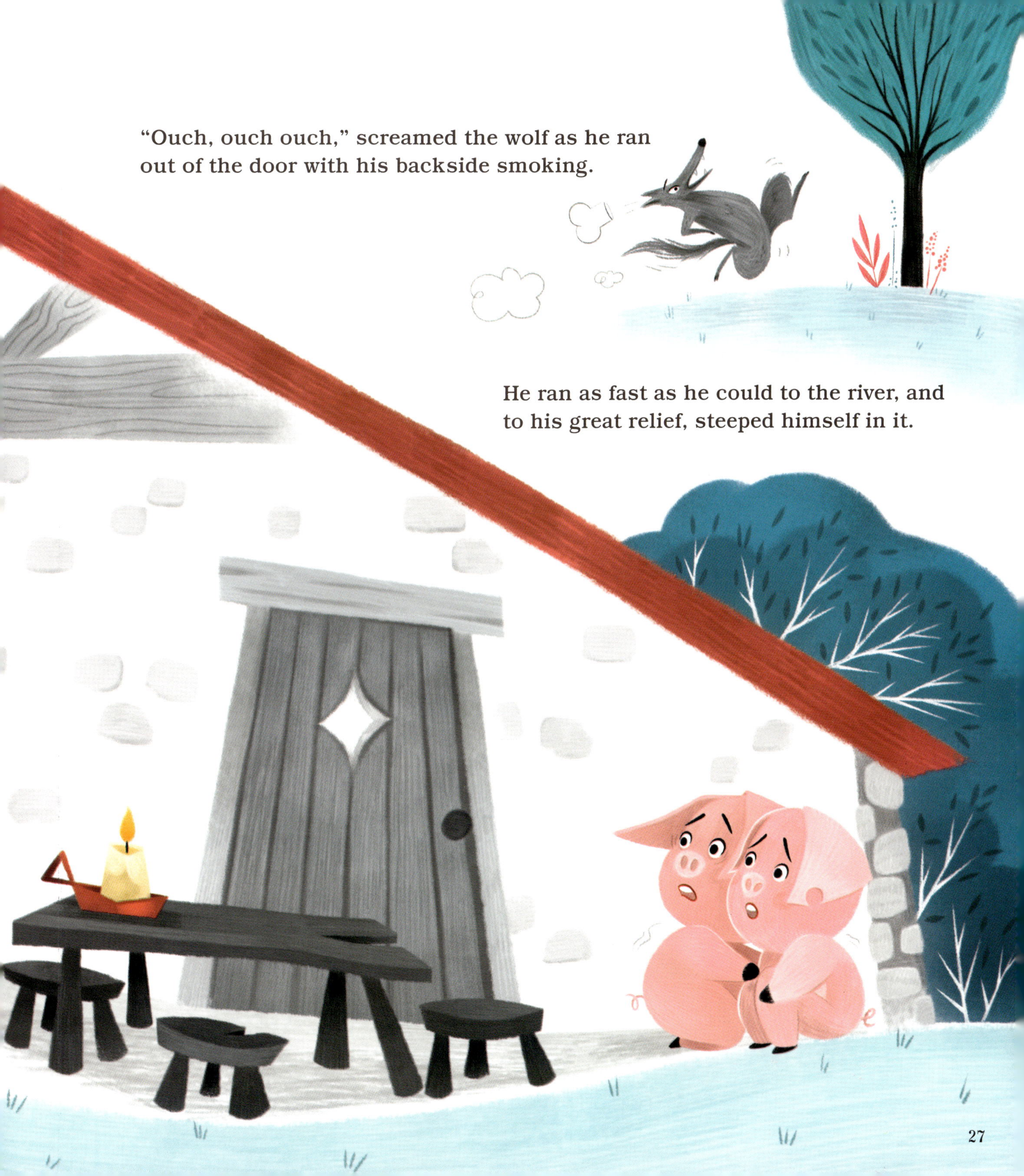

He ran as fast as he could to the river, and to his great relief, steeped himself in it.

Since that day, the three little pigs never saw the wolf again and lived happily together in the lovely stone house.

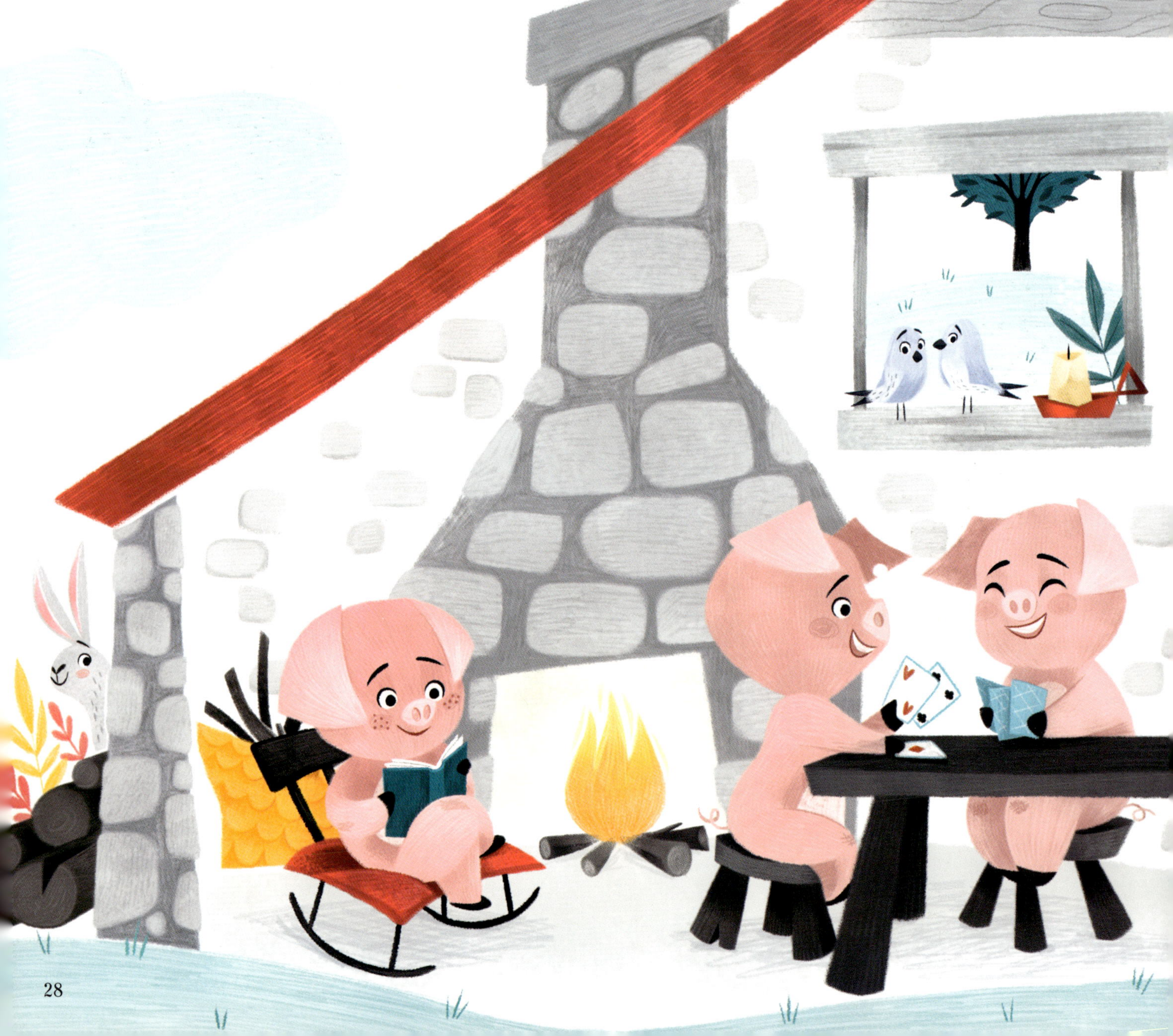

Relaxation

The story is finished. Now you shall relax.
◎ Choose a quiet place, with cushions and stuffed toys (or the blanket for instance)
◎ Dim the lights.
◎ Make yourself comfortable and read these texts to the child.
◎ Speak slowly and softly.
The relaxation proposed here is inspired by the Jacobson method, according to which, there exists a relation between emotions and muscular tension.

Preparation

"Lie down on your back. Keep your hands alongside your body, with your palms turned towards the sky. Don't move anymore. Smile softly as you close your eyes. Feel the weight of your entire body on the ground. We shall relax while playing a game called 'Tense and Relaxed'. This game shall make you aware of your hands. In the tale, the three little pigs have worked a lot with their hands. Thanks to the hands, they were able to touch the light straw, the flexible wicker and the hard stone."

Relaxation: Tense and Relaxed

"Draw your attention to the middle of your chest. Feel your heart beat. Now concentrate on your arms and hands that are extensions of your heart. Now concentrate on your hands while keeping your eyes closed. Feel the weight of your entire body on the ground. Clench your fists. Hold them tight. Then your fists become soft and they open. The fingers fall like wilted flowers. Try and notice the difference in the feeling when the fists are clenched, and when they are open... Do this three times. Feel your body resting. The entire body, the entire body..."

Waking up

Breathe deep. Now move your fingers. Move your toes. Stretch yourself. Yawn if you wish to. Gently turn your body to the side and sit up.

Rounding off

Stand up. With hands joined in front of your heart, greet yourself.

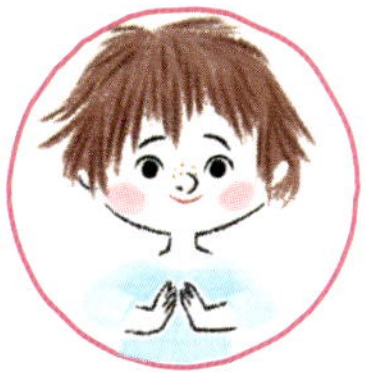

Postures

This tale shows that focus helps grow up well. While doing the postures associated with the tale, thanks to his body, the child identifies himself with the highs and lows our three little friends live through. Therefore, he acquires an alert and adaptable attitude so that he can grow up while building up a personality in harmony with others.

Listening

p. 2

Namasté or greetings

Benefit:
Helps focus.

5 breaths

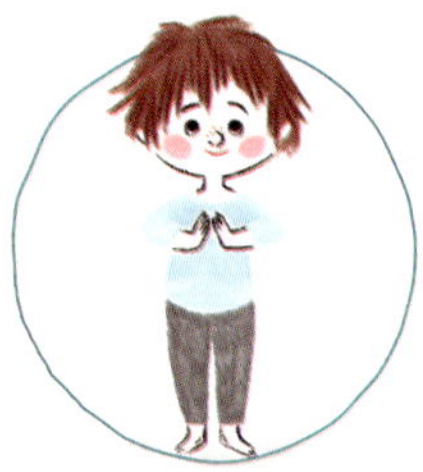

While standing, join your hands in front of your chest and bow your head.

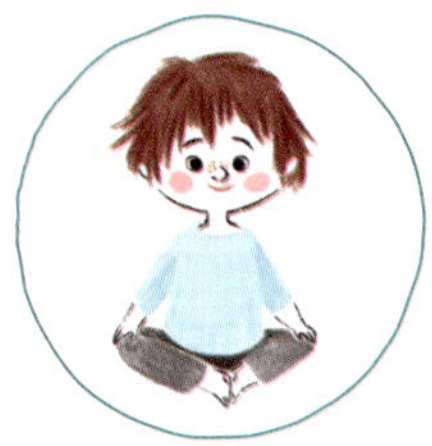

Sit down with your back straight and legs crossed.

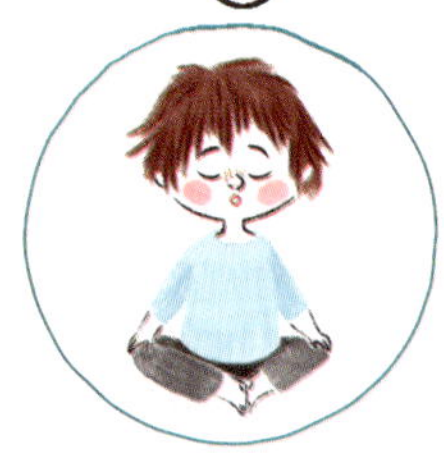

Breathe deep. Close your eyes. You are ready to listen to the story.

Relaxing legs

p. 5

Series of *Pawanmuktasanas* or the release of wind

Benefit: Good for balance and calm.

10 times

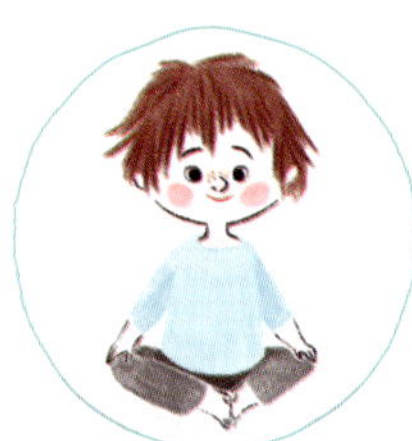

Sit with your back straight and legs crossed.

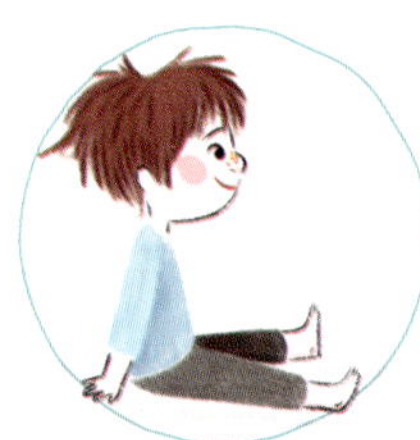

Place your legs slightly apart in a relaxed manner in front of you on the ground.

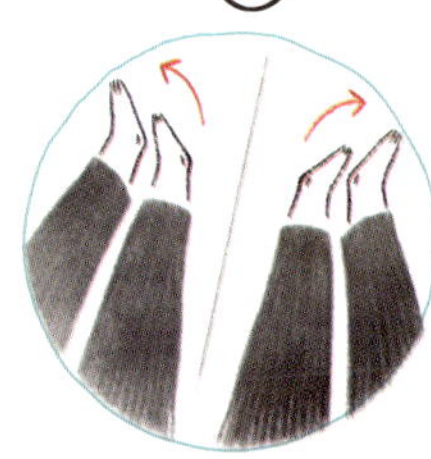

Turn your legs to one side, then the other while keeping your heels to the ground (movement of windscreen wipers).

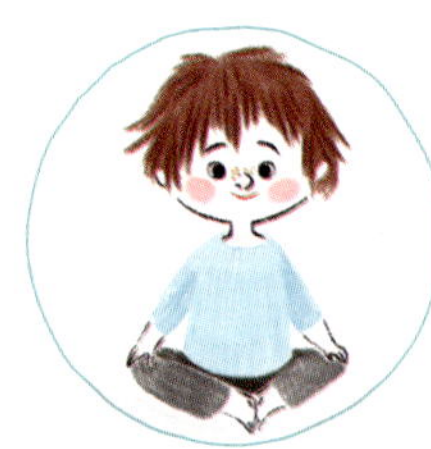

Get back to sitting cross-legged.

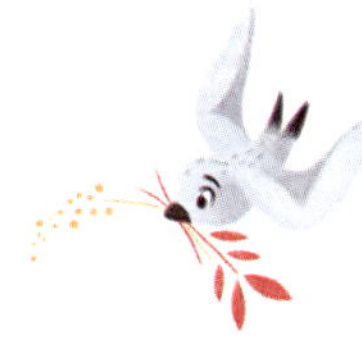

The straw house

p. 9

Simplified variation of *Upavishtha Konasana* or the posture of being seated at an angle
Benefit: Flexibility of the abductors.

4 times

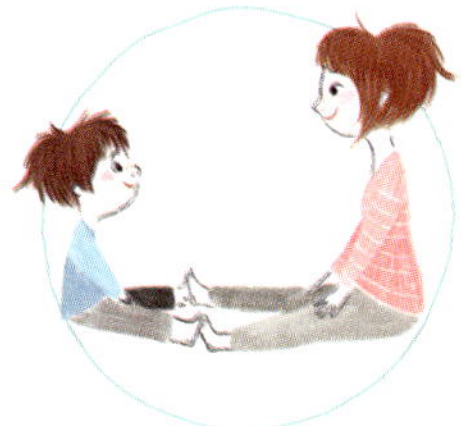

Sit facing each other. Place your legs in front of you and hold them apart them like a pair of scissors.

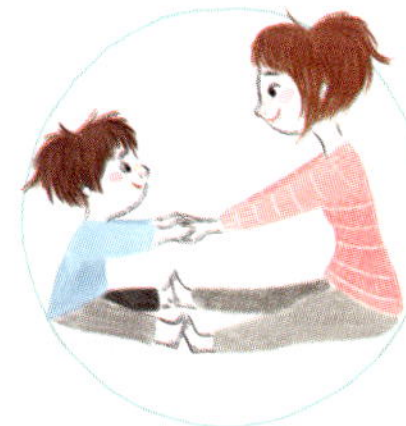

The soles of your feet must touch, and the adult must hold the child by his hands.

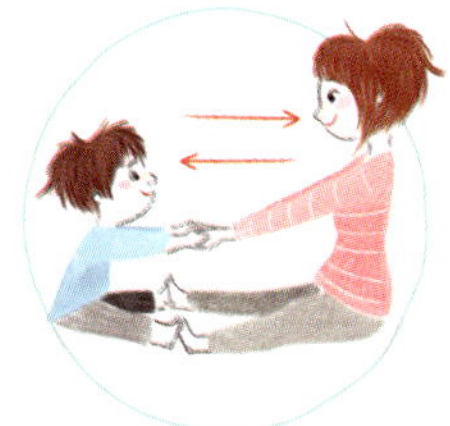

The child pulls the adult gently towards him. Then the movement is reversed.

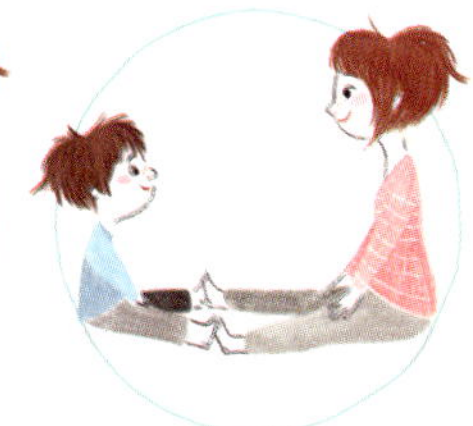

Let go of the hands gently and bring your legs back together.

The wicker house

p. 12

Adho Mukha Svanasana or the dog stretch
Benefit: Flexibility of the posterior muscle chain.

5 breaths

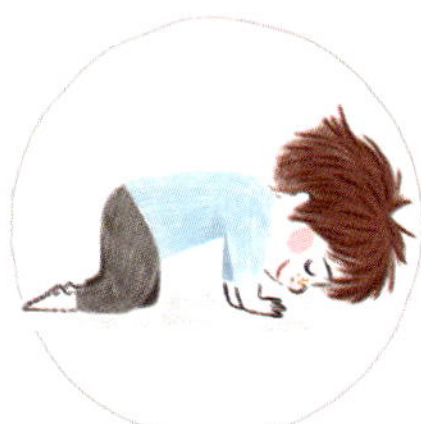

Get down on all fours.

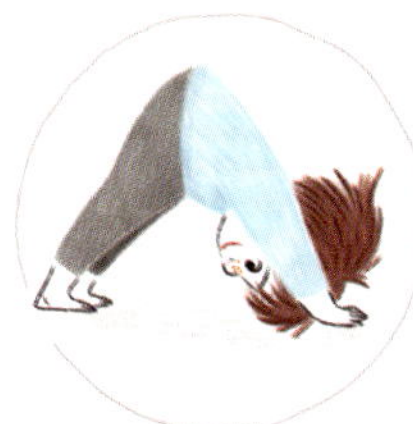

Lift the pelvis while pushing the ground with your hands. Your body forms a toboggan.

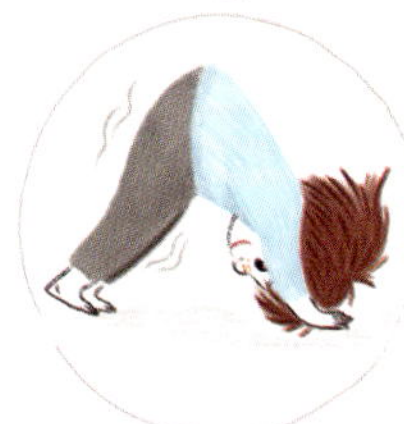

Enjoy moving the toboggan gentlly first with your legs, then with your hands.

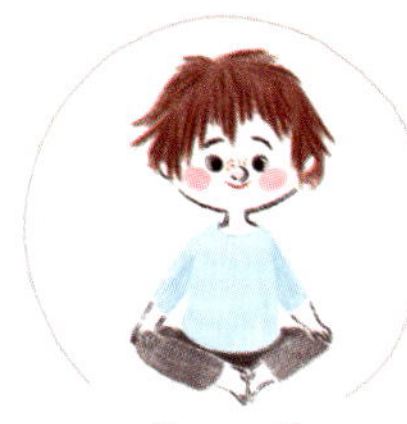

Sit down on your heels. Thereafter, sit cross-legged.

The roll

p. 15

Benefit: Self-massage of the spine.

4 times

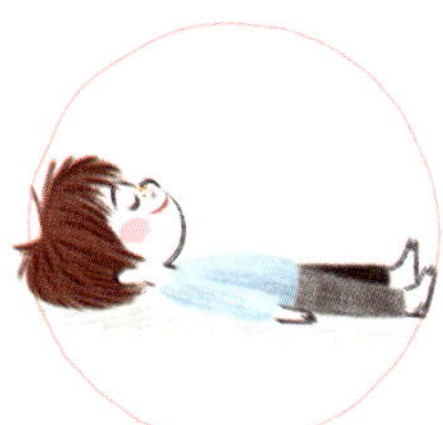

Lie down, with your back gently on the ground.

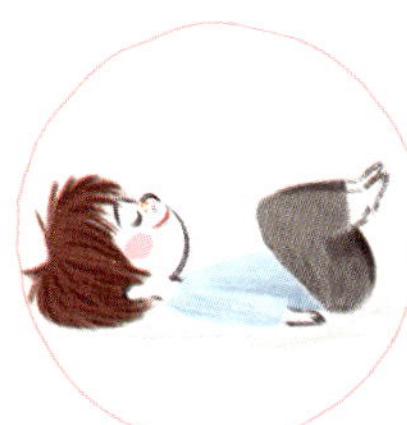

Fold your legs. Hold your knees above your chest.

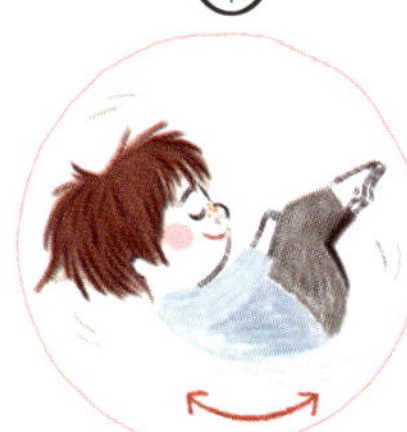

Hug your knees. Bend the spine and take in the chin. Rock gently from back to front.

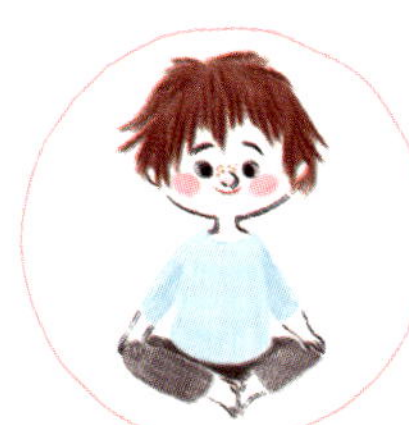

Get back to sitting cross-legged.

The chimney

p. 17

Simplified variation of *Dandasana* or the stick

Benefit: Awareness of the spine.

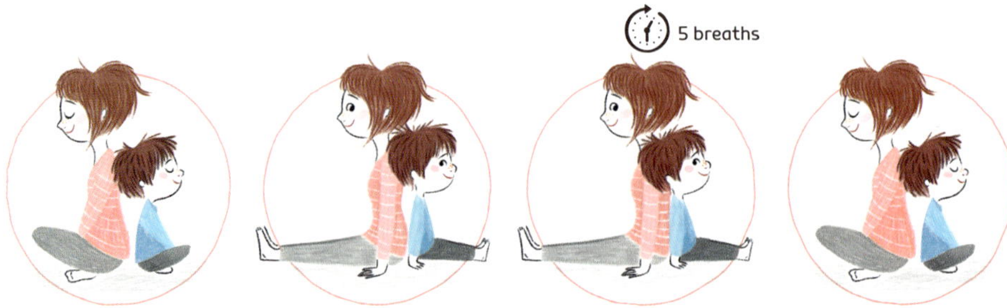

Sit cross-legged, back-to-back.

Join your legs and stretch them in front of you. Keep your arms by the side of the torso, and push the ground with your hands.

Adjust the posture so that the torsos form a rectangle.

Undo the posture and get back to sitting cross-legged.

The wolf blowing

p. 21

Initiation to *pranayama*

Benefits: Gets rid of tensions and opens oneself up to imagination.

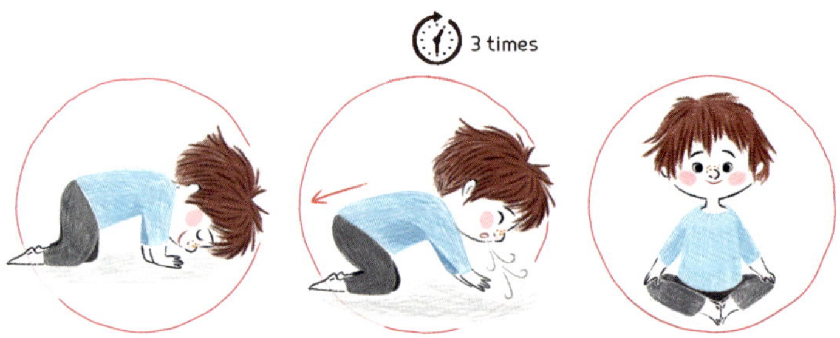

Sit on your heels, with your hands on either side of your body.

Place your hands on the ground so you are on all fours.

Move your pelvis back towards the heels. Take a deep breath through the nose and blow hard from the mouth.

Undo the posture and sit on your heels, then get back to sitting cross-legged.

The stone house

p. 25

Utkasana or the posture of the chair

Benefits: Force and stability.

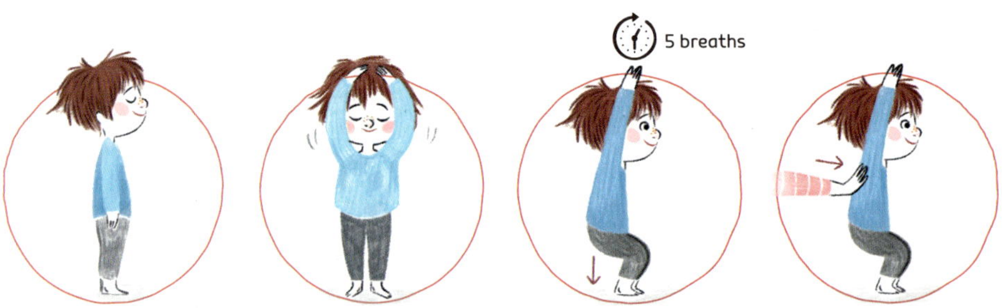

Stand so that your body is in a fine straight line.

Lift your hands from the front and join the palms above your head.

Flex your knees as though you are going to sit on a chair. Keep your back straight. Dig your heels into the ground.

The adult tests the solidness of the house by gently placing the hands against the back of the child. Then the child shall return to the initial posture and relax his body.